The Good
Skin Doctor

The Good Skin Doctor

A DERMATOLOGIST'S SURVIVAL GUIDE TO ACNE

TONY C CHU, FRCP
Senior Lecturer and Consultant Dermatologist
Imperial College of Science, Technology and Medicine
Hammersmith Hospital

ANNE LOVELL
Author, broadcaster and advice columnist, *Bella*

HarperCollins*Publishers*

While the authors of this work have made every effort to ensure that the information contained in this book is as accurate and up to date as possible at the time of publication, medical and pharmaceutical knowledge is constantly changing and the application of it to particular circumstances depends on many factors. Therefore it is recommended that readers always consult a qualified medical specialist for individual advice. This book should not be used as an alternative to seeking specialist medical advice, which should be sought before any action is taken. The authors and publishers cannot be held responsible for any errors and omissions that may be found in the text, or any actions that may be taken by a reader as a result of any reliance on the information contained in the text, which is taken entirely at the reader's own risk.

Thorsons
An Imprint of HarperCollins*Publishers*
77–85 Fulham Palace Road,
Hammersmith, London W6 8JB

Published by Thorsons 1999

10 9 8 7 6 5 4 3 2 1

A catalogue record for this book
is available from the British Library

ISBN 0 7225 3675 5

Printed and bound in Great Britain by
Caledonian International Book Manufacturing Ltd, Glasgow

Contents

Introduction

Acne is a disease – a disease that demands sympathetic management. It is a disease that scars not just the skin but also the psyche. It is a disease that is so common that it touches the lives of most people, but it is a disease that people in general know little about and about which there is enormous misunderstanding. Acne is also a stigma that sufferers must bear – something to be ashamed of, something to be ridiculed about.

As a former sufferer himself, Dr Tony Chu is only too well aware of the problems of living with and growing up with acne. As a patient he encountered ignorance about the disease and lack of sympathy from his physicians. As a dermatologist he was confronted with the scale of the problem, the suffering that acne caused and the joy of successfully treating patients. Recognizing the hurdles that confront the acne sufferer, and the lack of information and the support that they need, he founded the Acne Support Group in 1990.

The Acne Support Group is the only charity in the world devoted to the acne sufferer. Its short-term goals are to provide help, information and support for people who suffer from this disfiguring and depressing condition. The long-term goals are to change the public perception of acne from something to laugh at and to tease about, to an awareness of a disease that needs prompt and successful treatment, to help future generations avoid the physical and emotional scars.

The Group now has a membership of over 6,000 people in the UK. It aims to help members gain access to better treatment and offers a range of information sheets on various acne treatments, individual support and advice and a growing number of related services. This book was commissioned as a further resource for anyone for whom acne is a problem, and gathers together all the most up-to-date information and advice about living, coping and overcoming acne.

It has been written by Dr Chu, with Anne Lovell, advice columnist for *Bella* magazine, and a Board member of the Acne Support Group.

Anne Lovell:
One Sunday afternoon in the Spring of 1990, I caught a mention of the word 'acne' on the BBC TV programme The Clothes Show. *I heard that a support group for people who suffered from acne was being formed and I grabbed a pen to write down the information. The previous week I had received a letter to my column in* Bella *magazine, from a man who had reached desperation stage in his efforts to control his skin condition. He so hated the way he looked that he had taken down all the mirrors in his home. His letter had worried me, and suddenly here was something positive and hopeful I*

*could tell him about. I tracked down the Acne Support Group, told
my reader about it, and published the Group's address in my column.
I was invited to the first press conference to launch the ASG in 1992
– and joined the Board in 1994. As a sufferer of rosacea, another
common skin condition, at one time referred to as 'adult acne', I also
have a personal interest and involvement.*

Throughout the book, the medical aspects of acne are
described and discussed by Dr Chu, while non-medical areas
have been dealt with by Anne Lovell.

1

Understanding Acne

To understand acne and how you develop it, you need to understand the basic structure of the skin. In this first section, therefore, I will describe the skin and point out the parts of the skin involved in the process that leads to the development of acne.

The Structure of Normal Skin

If you look at the skin in cross-section under the microscope, you can see that it is composed of two parts (Figure 1). The upper part is called the *epidermis* and is composed of skin cells, or *keratinocytes*. These cells continually divide and, as they grow, they mature. As they reach the surface of the skin

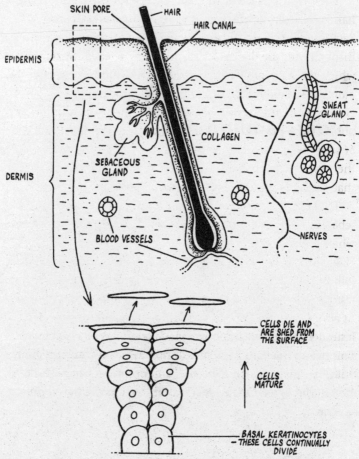

Figure 1

they flatten, die and are then shed from the surface of the skin. The deeper part of the skin is called the *dermis* and is composed mainly of *collagen*, which supports the epidermis. Within the collagen are the nerves, blood vessels and other structures that comprise the skin.

The whole surface of the skin, except for the palms of the hands and soles of the feet, is covered in small skin pores. Each pore is the entrance of a small, flexible tube that runs through into the dermis and represents the canal through which the hairs grow to the surface. Over most of the skin the hairs are so small that they are virtually invisible, or may not even grow to the surface of the skin. In the scalp, arm-pits and pubic area in men and women, and beard area, chest and back of some men, the hairs become coarser and longer and are, therefore, visible. Each hair canal is associated with a gland that produces oil, called the *sebaceous gland*.

The unit, consisting of the hair canal, the tiny hair and the sebaceous gland, is what we call the *pilosebaceous follicle*: this is where acne occurs.

Before puberty, everything is very quiet in the pilosebaceous follicle, but once you reach puberty the male hormone, testosterone – produced in women in the adrenal glands (which sit above the kidneys) and in the ovaries, and in men from the testes – activates the sebaceous gland, which then produces oil. This oil, or *sebum*, is pumped into the hair canal and from there onto the surface of the skin, where it lubricates the hair and the skin. This is a totally normal part of growing up and happens in everybody.

The Development of Acne

When you develop acne it is rather like a biological switch being switched on. We do not fully understand it but we know that the switch is switched on in most people by fluxes in hormone levels around the time of puberty. It may be switched on later in life by stress – this is the commonest cause of first-time acne in women in their mid- or late twenties. This 'maturity onset acne' was first recognized in the US in businesswomen who were climbing the corporate ladder. Because of their acne, many of these women gave up their jobs. We have recognized this type of acne in the UK over the last few years. Indeed, many acne sufferers find that their acne flares up when they are under stress – during exam times or when a relationship breaks up.

The switch that turns acne on turns off spontaneously in 70 per cent of sufferers after four or five years, which gives rise to the myth that everybody grows out of acne. **NOT EVERY-BODY 'GROWS OUT' OF ACNE.** Thirty per cent of people have acne that persists for longer than this period, and it may persist well through into their fifties and sixties. The oldest patient to be referred to me with acne was 81 years old, and she had had acne since she was 15 years of age. She is very fed up with people telling her she will grow out of it!

Figures on the incidence of acne are not readily available, but more than 80 per cent of adolescents develop acne. At the age of 40 years of age, the incidence is 1 per cent in men and 5 per cent in women, so there are a lot of older people with acne in the community.

As well as spontaneously switching off, the switch can also be switched off by effective treatment – and once it is switched off, it is quite possible that it will not switch on again. This is the rationale behind the treatments that we use in acne.

When the switch switches on, the first abnormality that occurs is that the oil gland becomes overly sensitive to the male hormone present. It is important to remember that in most people the problem is not that excess male hormone is being produced, it is just that the oil gland becomes over-sensitive to the male hormone present. **ACNE IS NOT A**

HORMONAL DISEASE. Increased male hormone levels are never found in men with acne. In some women the hormone levels can be abnormal, and this may be reflected by abnormalities in the menstrual cycle. In most women this does not influence treatment.

With the increased sensitivity of the gland to the male hormone, more oil is produced in the follicle and this leads to greasy skin, which is the hallmark of the acne sufferer (Figure 2). This in itself is not a problem and is not something that we can readily treat, particularly in men. Oil production tends to remain high throughout life and certainly until the mid- to late seventies, when the oil gland starts to wear out and produce less oil. This does have advantages, in that people with oily skin tend to age better and do not require excessive amounts of moisturizing creams, which a lot of people need to use as they get older.

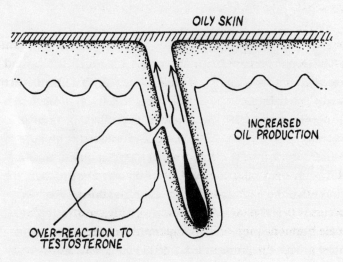

Figure 2

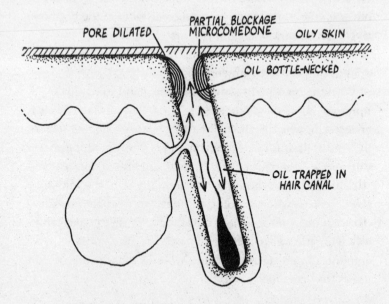

PORE DILATED
PARTIAL BLOCKAGE
MICROCOMEDONE
OILY SKIN
OIL BOTTLE-NECKED
OIL TRAPPED IN
HAIR CANAL

Figure 3

The second abnormality that occurs in the skin is the most important one, and this is a change in the cells that line the hair canals. The hair canals are flexible tubes which run through into the deeper layers of the skin. These tubes are lined by normal skin cells. As in the epidermis, these cells continually grow, mature and eventually die and, when they die, they normally float off into the oil stream and are taken onto the surface of the skin so that the hair canal remains clean and open. When you develop acne, however, these cells change and, instead of floating off when they die, they become very sticky and adhere to the inside of the canal. Over a period of months and years these dead cells build up and cause a partial blockage in the hair canal (Figure 3). This partial blockage is called a *microcomedone* and is the basic abnormality in the skin that leads to blackheads, whiteheads and then, eventually, inflammatory spots, papules, pustules and cysts of acne.

What causes this change in the growth of the cells within the hair canal is not fully understood, but some people feel that it is due to a change in the constituents of the oil being produced by the sebaceous gland.

The immediate impact of having this partial blockage in the hair canal is that the flexible tube dilates in response to the partial blockage and this makes the skin pores bigger, leading to the coarse complexion that is typical of the acne sufferer. If the blockage is close to the surface then you can see pigment in it, and it is this pigment – and not dirt – that represents the 'black' of the blackhead.

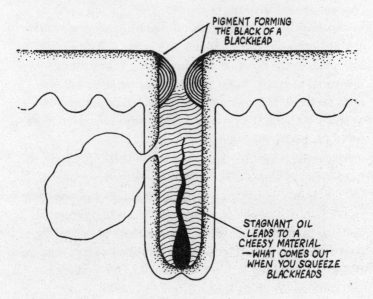

PIGMENT FORMING THE BLACK OF A BLACKHEAD

STAGNANT OIL LEADS TO A CHEESY MATERIAL —WHAT COMES OUT WHEN YOU SQUEEZE BLACKHEADS

Figure 4

If the blockage is deep in the skin, this just pushes the skin up slightly as a small bump in the skin and gives the skin in the acne sufferer its characteristic slightly bumpy, rough feeling. Deep in the skin the partial blockage restricts the flow of oil onto the surface; some of the oil is, therefore, diverted down into the deeper part of the hair canal, where it stagnates. Water is absorbed into the deeper part of the skin and this leaves a cheesy material which is what you squeeze out when you squeeze blackheads (Figure 4).

Periodically the partial blockage, or microcomedone, seals completely. This may be the result of the age of the blockage, but may also be the result of sweating, as sweat can be absorbed into the hair canal and cause the partial blockage to swell. In women the blockage can be affected by hormone changes around the time of menstruation. As you come up to your period, levels of the female hormone oestrogen, which counteracts the male hormone testosterone, fall precipitously. This leads to the eventual shedding of the womb lining and menstrual bleeding. As the female hormone levels fall, the male hormone becomes more dominant. This in turn can lead to spot formation. This is why a lot of women develop more spots just before their period.

When the partial blockage seals the follicle completely, oil cannot escape onto the surface and therefore accumulates under the skin, blowing up the hair canal rather like a small balloon under the skin (Figure 5). This leads to pressure building up in the skin, which you are aware of as tingling or pain although you can see nothing on the surface of the skin that may be causing it. You know that a spot is coming but you can't see anything there.

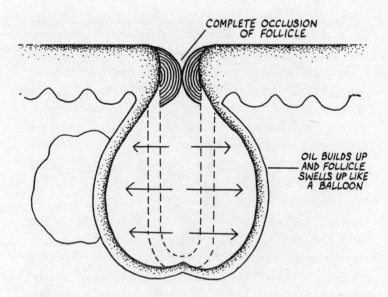

COMPLETE OCCLUSION
OF FOLLICLE

OIL BUILDS UP
AND FOLLICLE
SWELLS UP LIKE
A BALLOON

Figure 5

In all hair canals, bacteria are present. These are normal residents within the hair canal and are present in everybody, whether you have spots or not. As the oil accumulates in the follicle, these bacteria start to multiply and produce chemicals that will lead to inflammation. The whole area becomes inflamed and this leads to the first inflammatory spot of acne, which is a red spot or *papule*. How exactly the inflammation is generated is not fully understood, but this may in part be related to chemicals produced by the bacteria themselves, and also to the breakdown of oil in the sebum into inflammatory chemicals. Eventually, as part of the healing process the body recruits white blood cells into the follicle, which kill the bacteria, produce more inflammation and generate pus (Figure 6).

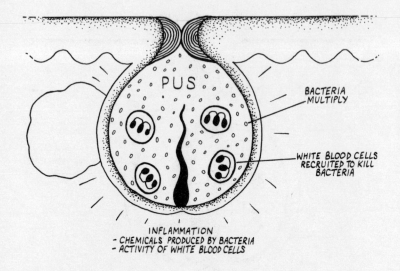

PUS

BACTERIA
MULTIPLY

WHITE BLOOD CELLS
RECRUITED TO KILL
BACTERIA

INFLAMMATION
- CHEMICALS PRODUCED BY BACTERIA
- ACTIVITY OF WHITE BLOOD CELLS

Figure 6

As the pus develops it then points through the hair canal to the surface and eventually bursts onto the surface, carrying the blockage with it – and everything starts all over again (Figure 7).

If the inflammation is very deep in the hair canal, the pus may not be able to point to the surface and escape. This leads to a deep sore lump in the skin which takes several weeks to go down. If the inflammation is particularly severe and deep in the hair canal, instead of bursting onto the surface the pus can burst inwards into the deeper part of the skin, which will lead to deeper inflammation with the risk of scarring. This is the main danger also in squeezing spots, as if you squeeze a spot there is a danger that the pus will burst inwards rather than outwards, once again leading to deep inflammation and eventual scarring.

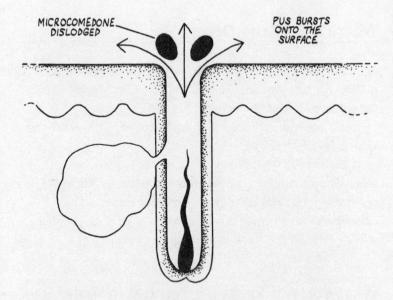

Figure 7

As some spots develop, the inflammation within the hair canal can be severe enough that part of the hair canal becomes detached; this then rounds up deeper in the skin rather like a flattened balloon, still with the oil gland attached. This acts as a focus for infection and inflammation, and when these hair canals become inflamed, the inflammation is much deeper. As there is no easy access to the surface of the skin, the spots come up as painful, deep spots that do not come to a head and usually take several weeks to go down again. The spot then recurs periodically. These are the cysts that occasionally occur in acne.

Where Does Acne Occur?

Acne can occur anywhere on the body where pilosebaceous follicles are present – that is, over the whole body apart from the palms of the hands and soles of the feet. In one patient I treated, his acne extended from his forehead to his wrists and ankles. Luckily this is very rare!

The commonest sites to get acne are the face and neck, followed by chest, back, upper arms and buttocks. The spots occur where the sebaceous glands are most active, and although in most people this is on the face, in some people it may be only on the chest, back or upper arms.

What Sorts of Spots Do You Get in Acne?

The clinical lesions of acne are the non-inflammatory spots or the blackheads and the whiteheads, and then the inflammatory spots which are the red papules, and then pustules and cysts. When scarring occurs in the skin this can be either soft-pitted scarring due to loss of part of the dermis, with the skin dimpling into it, or hard-pitted scarring, where the epidermis of the skin is caught up by the scar tissue and pulled deep into the skin, leading to a deep pit.

In some people, particularly on the chest and back, thick scars or *keloids* may occur as the result of acne spots. These scars are quite tender or itchy, they are hard and raised from the surface of the skin and initially are quite red. They often grow with time and can reach several centimetres in diameter. These may be the result of even quite trivial acne spots.

Conclusion

Acne is a chronic inflammatory condition in the skin which is caused by an abnormal response in the skin to normal levels of the male hormone, testosterone. Although related to hormones, in most people acne is not caused by an abnormality in the hormones. The key abnormalities that occur in the skin are:

- increased oil production
- partial blockage in the hair canal which leads to the development of the non-inflammatory blackheads and whiteheads
- eventually, the complete blockage of the hair canal which allows oil to accumulate, with growth of bacteria that are normally present in the skin, resulting in inflammation and giving rise to the inflammatory lesions of acne – the red papule, the pustule and the cyst.

The bacteria that are primarily implicated in the inflammation that occurs in acne are called *Propionibacterium acnes*. These bacteria are present in everybody's skin, but the abnormalities that occur in the acne sufferer allow the bacteria to cause inflammation in the skin.

2

Dispelling the Myths
Around Acne

One reason that acne sufferers feel so bad about their acne
is because of all the myths that surround acne. Most of these
firmly point an accusing finger at the sufferer as in some way
causing their acne by what they eat, how they wash and the
sort of person they are. It is very important to remember that
acne is a chronic inflammatory disease of the skin which is not
caused by anything that you do or don't do. It is a specific
disease and needs to be treated properly. It can be caused or
made worse if you are taking certain drugs for other medical
conditions, and can be made worse by certain makeup (*see
Chapter 9*).

What Myths Are Common in Acne?

1 Acne Is a Teenage Disease

WRONG!

Although the majority of people who develop acne do so around puberty and adolescence, acne is by no means only a disease of adolescence. There is a well-recognized population of older women in their mid- to late twenties or early thirties who develop acne for the first time. This population was first recognized in the US, but I see a lot of patients who develop acne at this time in their lives. In the majority of these patients it seems to be stress-related and usually occurs in young businesswomen who have very demanding jobs. Although acne will subside spontaneously after four or five years in 70 per cent of people, it can and does persist in a further 30 per cent of people well into adult life. The incidence of acne at 40 years of age is 1 per cent in men and 5 per cent in women. This means that there are a lot of people in their forties who still suffer quite badly with acne and require treatment.

While on holiday in Cyprus in October of 1997, I became very bored on the beach and so took a clipboard around the beach to do an acne survey. There were mainly older people there, in their forties and fifties, and on that beach at least 60 per cent of people had acne that needed treatment. Most of this was on the back and chest. This was an eye-opening experience for me – and nearly got me arrested!

Acne can persist well into old age and I have a number of patients in their sixties, seventies and even eighties who still have active acne. Acne is, therefore, not merely a teenage occurrence; it can affect you at any time in your life and can be apersistent problem through the whole of your adult life, unless it is treated properly.

2 Acne Is Caused by Eating Fatty Foods and Chocolate

WRONG!

A number of letters that I get from acne sufferers start with the phrase, 'I eat a very healthy diet and I don't eat fatty foods and I don't eat chocolate.' A number of doctors also give advice to patients to stop eating chocolate and not to eat fried food. Do fried foods and chocolate cause acne? Of course not!

There is a very simplistic concept: acne is associated with an oily skin, so it can be caused by eating too much oil which leaks onto the surface of the skin. Dietary oil has *no* impact on oil production in the skin. You could eat a bucket of blubber and your skin's oil production would not change at all. The only factors that influence oil production in the skin are the male hormone testosterone and temperature. In hot environments, oil production in the skin increases. That is why your skin often feels greasier when it is hot or when you go on holiday to a hot country.

There have been very large studies which have looked at diet in acne, particularly in the US, which have shown no correlation between diet and acne. It is bad enough having acne, without being told that you can't go to McDonald's with your friends and that you can't eat chocolate. There are, however, some patients who do develop worsening of their condition when they eat chocolate or fatty foods, and obviously they should avoid whatever does make their skin flare up. These people, however, really are the minority; most people with acne can eat whatever they like without affecting their acne. The idea that you can't is really just another stick for people to beat you with because you've got acne and to make you feel bad about yourself.

It is always best when you look at a chronic disease to take a holistic approach towards treatment, and therefore a good balanced diet should be part of your management of acne. However, this does not mean that you need to avoid foods which you enjoy and foods which you like.

3 Acne Is Caused by Too Much or Too Little Sex

WRONG!

Because the majority of people who develop acne tend to be adolescents, the great unspoken fear is that it is all wrapped up with sex. Have I got acne because I haven't had sex? Have I got it because I've had too much sex? Because I masturbate?

This is yet another myth to make you feel bad about yourself and that you are in some way causing the problem by what you do and who you are. The simple answer is that sex has no part to play in acne.

Acne is caused by an abnormal response in the skin to the male hormone testosterone. In the vast majority of patients this is not because of an abnormal level of the male hormone in the blood and certainly has nothing to do with whether you have sex, whether you don't have sex or whether you masturbate.

4 Acne Is Caused by Poor Cleanliness

WRONG!

This once again harks back to the image that society has of the acne sufferer as being a dirty, greasy-skinned, pimply youth, who is generally not a nice person. Are spots caused by failure to wash the skin? Of course not! Most patients with acne tend to overdo washing of their skin. This is partly because the skin is oily, so many acne sufferers will wash their skin several times a day to remove the oil. This, of course, is not good for the skin as it tends to dry out the top layers of the skin. This in turn can make the skin overly sensitive, too sensitive for the use of many of the acne creams and lotions which are very effective in this disease.

A lot of the acne washes on the market can also cause drying of the skin. My normal recommendation is that people should wash their skin twice a day with a simple soap. In those people who have rather delicate skin which may become irritated by the use of soap, try a soapless cleansing bar such as that produced by Neutrogena®, or a soap for sensitive skin, such as Dove® soap.

It is important, however, not to over-wash the skin as this can make the skin too sensitive and too dry.

5 Acne Will Get Better If You Get Pregnant

WRONG!

I have had a number of letters from patients which have said that their acne gets better when they are pregnant, or who have been told by their doctor that their acne will get better when they become pregnant. Pregnancy is not, however, a particularly good treatment for acne!

Some women certainly improve when they become pregnant; this is probably related to the increase in female hormones that occurs during pregnancy, which suppresses the male hormone and therefore leads to an improvement in their acne. However, some women develop acne for the first time when they are pregnant, and some women may develop worsening of their acne when they become pregnant; there is certainly no way of predicting which way acne will go during pregnancy and I would certainly not rely on pregnancy to improve acne.

6 Acne Is Something You Will Grow Out Of

WRONG!

This statement, I think, is one of the worst that is ever used in medicine. No patient should ever be told that they will 'grow out of' their acne. This to me seems to be a way for physicians to get out of the responsibility of treating acne by telling patients to leave it to nature. Acne does indeed get better in about 70 per cent of patients after four or five years – but during these four or five years patients with acne may suffer enormously because of it. They may develop significant scarring of the skin, and scarring of the skin is permanent. They may also develop significant psychological scarring because of their acne.

Always remember that at least 30 per cent of people who develop acne do *not* grow out of it in four or five years; it can persist right the way through into adult life. It is very important, therefore, to start the treatment of acne as soon as possible, to prevent permanent scarring of the skin and to try to switch off the mechanism of acne formation as quickly as possible, so that you don't have to suffer from it any longer than is necessary.

7 If You Have a Pusy Spot, You Have Got to Squeeze It

WRONG!

Spot-squeezing is almost a national pastime, and I find it very difficult to persuade my patients not to squeeze their spots. There is a great danger in squeezing spots – you can actually cause more damage to the skin and this could ultimately lead to permanent scarring of the skin. Never squeeze blackheads with your fingers. If you look at a blackhead, it is essentially a solid lump of grease that has developed in the hair canal and has a pigmented top to it, which is the black of the blackhead. By squeezing the skin, it is possible to squeeze a lot of the grease out – but there is also a danger that some of the grease can be forced deeper into the skin, where it can damage the deeper structures of the hair canal and then lead to inflammation and the development of a deep spot (Figures 8 and 9).

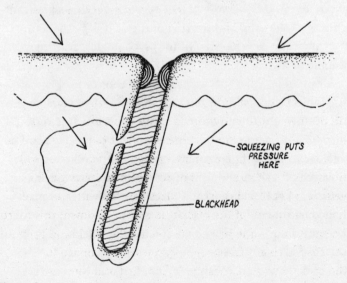

SQUEEZING PUTS PRESSURE HERE

BLACKHEAD

Figure 8

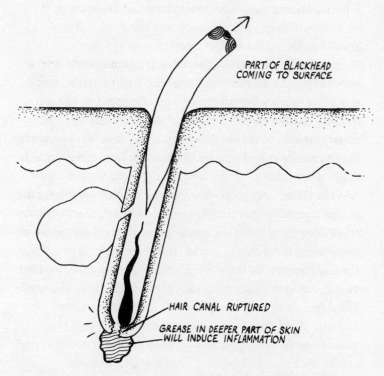

PART OF BLACKHEAD
COMING TO SURFACE

HAIR CANAL RUPTURED

GREASE IN DEEPER PART OF SKIN
WILL INDUCE INFLAMMATION

Figure 9

If you have a lot of blackheads and you really want to get rid of them quickly, invest in a comedone spoon from your local pharmacist or The Body Shop®. A comedone spoon is a very small, spoon-shaped piece of metal which has a small hole drilled in one end. It is inexpensive and very good at getting rid of blackheads. You place the end with the small hole over the top of the blackhead and push down; this exerts pressure around the hair canal, forcing the blackhead up from the base so that it can be removed without damage to the underlying skin. Wash your skin first and then use the comedone spoon carefully.

Recently, adhesive comedone removers have become available which can help in removing blackheads. These are sold as Biore Pore Perfect Deep Cleansing Strip® and Oxy Blackout®. The principle behind this is that a quickly drying glue is applied to the skin and then squeezed into the mouth of the hair canal using a strip of tape. You allow the glue to dry for a few minutes and then carefully pull the tape off. When you look at the undersurface of the tape you can see the microcomedones and the solidified oil projecting from the surface like tacks (*for further details see Chapter 4*).

What about pusy spots? Very few people will be willing to go out in public with a large pusy spot on their face or nose. I have, therefore, given up telling my patients not to squeeze pusy spots – but I do explain to them how to do it properly. The most important thing to remember is that unless you can see pus, the spot is almost certainly not ready to be squeezed – and if you do squeeze it you could cause damage deep in the skin that could lead eventually to scarring. It is very much better to leave pusy spots to resolve by themselves, as this will lead to the minimum amount of scarring in the skin.

However, if you develop a pusy spot and you cannot face going out with it, carefully wash your hands, sterilize a pin or a needle in a flame and let it cool down, carefully puncture the skin over the collection of pus, then gently squeeze the spot to remove the pus. Do not squeeze until you see blood – if you see blood, it means you have damaged the little blood vessels around the hair root and this could potentially lead to scarring. There is no need to see blood coming through after the pus. This is another common myth, that you have to see blood to be sure you have washed out all the germs from the skin. This is nonsense. The pus that you are removing from the skin has no live bacteria in it; these have all been killed by the white blood cells. You are, therefore, only removing a collection of dead bacteria and white blood cells that would eventually have burst onto the surface. You need to be very gentle in removing the pus and nothing more.

The Facts About Acne

1 Acne is a chronic inflammatory disease of the skin which is not caused by anything you have done, either to yourself or to your skin.

2 Acne tends to run in families – if you have one parent who had severe acne, your chances of developing bad acne are higher. Also if you have a parent who has had persistent acne, your chances of developing persistent acne are higher.

3 Acne will resolve spontaneously in 70 per cent of people after four or five years, but there is no way of predicting whose will resolve after four or five years and whose will continue to cause problems for the next 30 or 40 years.

4 Acne should be treated as early as possible, to prevent scarring of the skin and to limit the embarrassment and psychological side-effects that the disease causes.

5 Acne is *not* caused by the food you eat and, in particular, it is not caused by eating fatty foods or chocolate.

6 Acne is *not* related to sex, either too much or too little, or to masturbation.

7 Acne does *not* necessarily get better during pregnancy. In some women it can get worse during pregnancy.

8 Acne is *not* caused by poor hygiene of the skin. The skin should be washed regularly twice a day. Excess washing of the skin can cause problems with drying of the skin.

9 Acne spots should *not* be squeezed. If you have blackheads, use a comedone spoon or tape remover; if you have a pusy spot and you have to squeeze the spot, use the instructions given above and never squeeze until you see blood.

3

Treating Your Acne

As you will have read in Chapter 2, acne is a condition that will spontaneously settle after four or five years in up to 70 per cent of people. There is no way, however, of predicting how bad acne can get in those four to five years, or whose acne will or won't settle spontaneously in those four or five years.

Acne can and does cause enormous suffering for those who are affected by it, and needs to be treated as soon as possible. Early treatment should limit the severity of acne and prevent the physical and psychological scarring that can be caused by acne. It is, however, up to you to treat your acne or get treatment for it.

Each patient with acne is different and will respond slightly differently to any given treatment. Treatment should, therefore, be tailored to the patient: to the extent of their disease, to their skin type and how well or badly they tolerate the different treatments.

Mild Acne

If your acne is mild, your first port of call should be your local pharmacist to find out what he or she would recommend. In Chapter 4 I have listed the treatments that you can buy over the counter and the types of acne they are effective in. Do remember that most of the products sold at the pharmacist for acne are ranges of treatment which will include the active anti-acne treatment as well as washes, lotions, cleansing pads, moisturizers, etc. which are not necessary to achieve a good result. They may suit your skin and help control your acne, but are not essential and will not suit all people.

The most important thing to remember is that acne treatments are not universally effective. If a treatment is not working for you, you must seek further advice.

In general, I would expect a 50 per cent improvement in acne after two months of treatment if the treatment is going to work for you. If you have achieved this result, continue the treatment until the acne is completely clear. If you have not achieved this result, take the next step and see your doctor for further advice.

Moderate-to-Severe Acne or Acne That Does Not Respond to Over-the-Counter Products

If you have moderate to severe acne, you are at risk of scarring and it is unlikely that you will respond well to products that you can buy over the counter. You should, therefore, make an appointment to see your doctor.

Dealing with Your Doctor

Your doctor is your vital link with the range of services and treatments available to you. Acne can be difficult to manage, and some more aggressive treatments cost a great deal of money. Doctors can be reluctant to refer you for expensive drugs, unless they are convinced you need them and they will work for you.

So it may well pay you to establish a good, working relationship with your doctor from the beginning of your consultation with him or her, so that you both feel you are able to communicate fairly with each other.

Doctors are people, like you and me, and they deserve to be treated with courtesy and civility as well as with informed assertiveness.

Doctors are also very busy people, so it is always advisable to have what you want to say prepared before your visit.

If you think you might feel too upset to concentrate, listen and respond, ask a family member or friend to come with you to the appointment.

Before Treatment Is Prescribed

To get the best from a visit to the doctor, think about what he or she might ask and have your answers ready. For example:

- How long has the condition been troubling you?
- What treatments have you already tried, for example over-the-counter products or other medication?

- Is it worse at certain times – before your period, when you're anxious, or as a reaction to foods or to cosmetics?

Being prepared will save time and frustration on both sides and provide the best diagnosis and treatment for you. Try not to let embarrassment hinder your description of the symptoms and, indeed, how you feel about yourself and acne. Even though doctors are only human, like you and me, they've probably heard more about things other people feel embarrassed about than most – and should be able to handle it!

Your emotional state is as important as your skin condition and you should be prepared to answer questions or to be frank about the way you feel, as much as about the details of your acne. You might be asked questions such as:

- Does your condition depress you sometimes/a great deal/always?
- Is your social life affected by your acne?
- Do you avoid school/college/work because of your acne?
- Do you feel that nobody understands how acne affects you/your lifestyle/your relationships?

Once your condition has been discussed, the doctor should prescribe medication which should clear, or at least control, your acne. Before you leave, make sure you are clear in your own mind about the following points:

- how to take or apply the medication
- how long it will be before an improvement might be expected to be noticeable
- what possible side-effects might be expected
- how long the course of treatment will last

- when you should schedule a follow-up appointment
- if this treatment proves unsuccessful – the further options
- when a referral to a dermatologist would be recommended.

Acne treatments require a considerable degree of patience –
from doctors – and more particularly from patients! It is
important to continue the course of treatment right through
to the end – unless side-effects become intolerable, in which
case this should be reported immediately and an alternative
prescription discussed.

Determination – and discipline – are essential requirements
for anyone who wants to achieve the best from their acne
treatment – and from their doctor.

Referral to the Dermatologist

In general, you need to be referred to a dermatologist by your
doctor. This is because your doctor must be kept informed of
treatment you are taking and will usually be asked to provide
any prescriptions for the drugs you need. In the UK, if you see a
dermatologist privately he or she cannot give you an NHS
prescription, only a private prescription. If you buy your anti-
acne drugs privately, they can be very expensive. If your doctor
has referred you, he/she will usually be happy to provide the
drugs you need on the NHS. Remember that most health
insurances will cover the cost of consultation with a dermatologist but not the cost of any drugs that are prescribed.

Patients, as such, cannot demand a referral to a hospital
dermatologist, this is done solely at the discretion of the
doctor. In the new NHS here in Britain, many doctors are
fund-holders, which means that they are allocated a sum of
money by the Government and from this they must pay for

their patients to be seen at the hospital. This should have no impact on referral of patients to the hospital if they need to be referred. It must, however, discourage hospital referral in some cases.

If you feel that your doctor is being unfair in not referring you to the hospital, discuss this with him or her, with documentation of how long you have had acne and how many treatments you have tried without success. If your doctor still refuses to refer you, you can make a complaint to the local Family Practitioners Association, which is the UK body that controls doctor activity.

4

Treatment for Acne – Preparations Applied to the Skin

What I have attempted in the following chapters is to give an overview of the treatments available, the way the treatments work, and some indication as to what to expect from your treatment.

Blackheads, Whiteheads and Comedonal Acne

Many patients with acne have a predominance of non-inflammatory spots. There is no redness or pain, just open pores, blackheads and whiteheads, giving the skin a rough appearance and feel. Occasional pusy spots may occur, but the main problem is the non-inflamed spots. The only effective treatments for this type of acne are:

- salicylic acid (aspirin) creams, gels and washes
- mechanical blackhead removers
- vitamin A creams, gels or lotions
- azelaic acid creams.

What Can I Buy Myself?

Only salicylic acid preparations and mechanical blackhead removers are available over the counter.

SALICYLIC ACID PREPARATIONS

Salicylic acid is present in gels, creams and washes. Most of these contain 2 per cent salicylic acid and are applied at night and washed off the next morning.

How Does It Work?

Salicylic acid is a *keratolytic*, which means that it dissolves dead skin cells. If you look at Chapter 1, you will see that it is a build-up of dead cells in the hair canal that leads to a build-up of oil and the development of non-inflammatory spots. The salicylic acid penetrates into the skin pore and helps to clean out some of these dead cells, allowing the oil to drain more freely onto the surface of the skin.

How Long Does It Take to Work?

Salicylic acid does not work quickly on non-inflamed acne spots. You will need to use it for several months before you see real benefits. Salicylic acid does help other treatments such as the vitamin A creams, and does make the skin feel less oily. As long as your skin tolerates it well, it is worth using these preparations as part of your skin cleansing regime.

Are There Any Side-effects?

In some people, salicylic acid can dry the skin and make it irritable. The use of a simple moisturizer is often sufficient to stop this, and the skin often becomes used to the salicylic acid after a week or two. In occasional users, an allergy to the salicylic acid can develop where the skin becomes red and very itchy. If this occurs you must stop the salicylic acid immediately and should not use it again.

MECHANICAL BLACKHEAD REMOVERS

These are available at the pharmacist and are certainly worth trying if you have a lot of blackheads. The principle was first put forward by an American dermatologist, Al Kligman, who developed the Exolift system®. This system is widely used in the US by dermatologists and beauticians, but has not really caught on in the UK.

Two products are currently available over the counter in the UK. Biore Pore Perfect Deep Cleansing Strip® and Oxy Blackout®.

How Does It Work?

The basic principle behind these blackhead removers is that a quick-drying resin or glue is applied to the affected area of skin, pressed into the skin pores by an impermeable tape, and allowed to dry. Once dry, the tape is carefully peeled off the skin and the blackheads, which have stuck to the tape, will come away.

How Long Does It Take to Work?

The treatment time depends on how much skin is being treated. The resin takes about 3 minutes to dry, and to do a small area of the skin, like the nose, can take a matter of 15 minutes or so. The blackheads will start to develop again, as this is not a treatment that stops blackheads from developing, but when used in conjunction with other treatment for comedones it can be very useful. The treatment can be repeated every two to four weeks depending on the response rate.

Are There Any Side-effects?

Directly after the treatment the skin can become red; this redness lasts about an hour or so. Some people may become allergic to the resin, which will cause a red itchy rash in the treated area a day or two after the treatment has been used. This will last about seven days and will leave the skin dry and scaly. If this occurs you cannot use the product again, as the allergic reaction will develop each time you use it.

What Can I Get from My Doctor?

Some forms of salicylic acid can be prescribed by your doctor. The majority of these are creams or solutions that the pharmacist will make up. A wash, containing 2 per cent salicylic acid, is commercially available. Known in the UK as Acnisal® wash, it is a good addition to any acne cleansing routine.

TOPICAL VITAMIN A DERIVATIVES

If salicylic acid by itself is not clearing the problem, or if you cannot use it, you should go to your doctor and ask for one of the vitamin A or retinoid preparations. There are three which can be obtained on prescription: Retin A® (also available under this name in the US), Isotrex® gel, and Differin® gel.

Retin A® (generic name tretinoin) is available in two strengths in the UK – 0.01 per cent and 0.025 per cent. There are gels, creams and lotions available, depending on your skin type.

Isotrex® gel is only available in one strength, containing 0.05 per cent isotretinoin, and only as a gel. (Not available in the US.)

Differin® gel contains 0.1 per cent adapalene in a gel formulation. (Not available in the US.)

If you have very greasy skin, gels or lotions are better than creams. If you have dry patches or a sensitive skin, a cream is better.

These preparations should be used once a day, in the evening after washing the skin. Use wherever you have problems – face, back, chest, arms, etc. – leave on overnight and wash off in the morning. Use on the whole affected area, not just on the spots you can see. Many of the blocked hair canals are so small that you cannot see them.

How Does It Work?

Vitamin A works by an effect on the way skin cells grow and mature. As you've read in Chapter 1, the build-up of dead skin cells in the hair canal is due to an abnormal growth of the skin cells lining the canal. Vitamin A normalizes growth of the skin cells and not only unseats existing partial blockages in the canal, but prevents new ones from developing (Figure 10). Vitamin A preparations are thus the treatment of choice in non-inflammatory acne, and also have a major role in the treatment of all types of acne by preventing the abnormality that allows spots to develop.

Vitamin A has one other major effect on the skin. It increases collagen production by the fibroblasts – cells in the structural part of the skin, or dermis, that make collagen. This is deposited just below the epidermis – the growing part of the skin – and produces a cushion that smoothes out wrinkles and can help to smooth out some superficial scars (Figure 11). The stronger

Figure 10

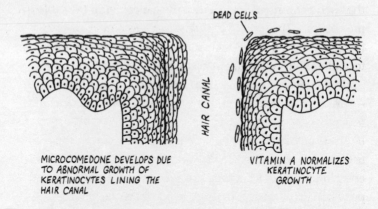

MICROCOMEDONE DEVELOPS DUE
TO ABNORMAL GROWTH OF
KERATINOCYTES LINING THE
HAIR CANAL

VITAMIN A NORMALIZES
KERATINOCYTE
GROWTH

vitamin A creams are best at doing this. The only one available
in the UK at the moment is Retinova® cream, which contains
0.05 per cent tretinoin but cannot be prescribed on the NHS,
only on private prescription.

How Long Does It Take to Work?

As with salicylic acid, the vitamin A preparations do not work
quickly. In the first two months you should notice an appreciable
change in the texture of the skin, with loss of the more obvious

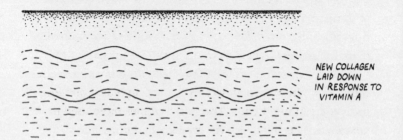

NEW COLLAGEN
LAID DOWN
IN RESPONSE TO
VITAMIN A

Figure 11

blackheads. With persistent use, the whiteheads should clear and the open pores should close down. Be patient with the vitamin A preparations. They will have little direct effect on pusy spots (apart from Differin® gel, which has some effect on the inflammatory spots), but will eventually prevent them from occurring.

Are There Any Side-effects?

Vitamin A can be very irritating to the skin. Isotrex® gel tends to be less irritating than Retin A®, but both preparations must be used with caution. Differin® gel, because of its anti-inflammatory effect, tends to be the best tolerated of all the vitamin A preparations, and tends to be the first of these agents that I prescribe.

You do not need to get irritation to get the benefits of the vitamin A. Start with Differin® gel, Isotrex® gel or the lower-strength Retin A®. The main cause of irritation is over-use, so be careful how much you use. A dollop about the size of a pea is enough to cover the whole face. Three to four times that amount will cover the back or chest. Apply it to the skin when it is perfectly dry – dry after washing, and then let the skin air dry for about 15 to 20 minutes before applying the preparation.

Always remember to wash the vitamin A off the skin the next morning. This is important, as if you leave it on the skin and then go out into the sunshine the skin can develop a marked sunburn reaction. If the skin becomes dry and scaly, use a moisturizer in the morning. If the skin becomes very sore, stop the vitamin A for a few days and then start again using it on alternate days to slowly build up your tolerance until you can use it daily. The skin becomes more used to vitamin A with time and will eventually not react to it.

Vitamin A when taken in tablet form can affect an unborn baby and cause abnormalities. For this reason, the makers of

Retin A®, Isotrex® gel and Differin® gel do not recommend the use of these products if you are a woman and thinking of having a baby or if you are pregnant. The actual amount of vitamin A that penetrates through the skin is minute, so in reality this is probably not a problem, but it is best to follow the manufacturers' advice.

Mild Inflammatory Acne

It is important to realize that even if you only have a few spots, this is still acne. It is also important to remember that it is impossible to predict whether these few pusy spots will eventually disappear with time or whether the problem will increase in severity, leaving you with a lot of deep-seated spots and possible scarring. I feel, therefore, that it is important that anyone with acne should have active treatment as soon as possible.

What Can I Buy Myself?

BENZOYL PEROXIDE

The main ingredient in most anti-acne preparations available over the counter is benzoyl peroxide. This is a very effective treatment for acne and should be regarded as the first line treatment of choice in mild acne. A list of common UK brand names is given in the table below. The creams or gels are available in different strengths – 2.5 per cent, 5 per cent and 10 per cent – and should be applied to the skin twice daily after washing the skin. If you have a lot of black- and whiteheads, use this with a salicylic acid preparation – see above.

Benzoyl Peroxide Preparations

Name of Product	Percentage of Benzoyl Peroxide
Acetoxyl® gel	2.5 per cent
Acnecide®	5 per cent
Benoxyl®	5 and 10 per cent
Benzagel®	5 per cent
Mediclear®	5 and 10 per cent
Nericur®	5 per cent
Oxy®	5 and 10 per cent
Panoxyl®	2.5, 5 and 10 per cent
Quinoderm®	5 and 10 per cent

Benzagel®, Oxy® and Panoxyl® are also sold in the US, as are the benzoyl peroxide preparations Ambi 10®, Ben-Aqua®, Benzac®, Brevoxyl®, Dermoxyl®, Fostex®, Peroxin®, Persagel® and Vanoxide®.

How Does It Work?
Benzoyl peroxide is an oxidizing agent. Its major use in industry is as a bleaching agent for flour. In the context of acne, benzoyl peroxide works because it kills the bacteria that cause the pusy, inflamed spots. As described in Chapter 1, the main bacteria that causes the inflamed spots of acne is *Propionibacterium acnes*. This is what we call an anaerobic bacterium, which means that it can only grow where there is no air – that is, in the hair canal. Benzoyl peroxide releases oxygen into the hair canal and thus kills the bacteria. It also penetrates right into the hair canal, which helps to prevent new spots from occurring.

How Long Does It Take to Work?

As with all treatments for the inflamed spots of acne, benzoyl peroxide does not work overnight. I usually expect at least a 50 per cent improvement in the spots in the first two months of treatment. If you have not achieved this then you are on the wrong treatment and should see your doctor to get something different. It is mainly the inflammatory spots, the red and pusy spots, that respond to benzoyl peroxide, but some larger blackheads will also clear.

Are There Any Side-effects?

Benzoyl peroxide is an oxidizing agent and can thus irritate the skin. You should use it sparingly, and if you have sensitive skin start at the 2.5 per cent strength and increase the strength after a few weeks. If you have normal skin you should be able to tolerate the 5 per cent strength and could increase to 10 per cent after a few weeks. If the skin becomes very red and scaly, stop the benzoyl peroxide for a few days and then increasing usage gradually. If the skin becomes dry, you can use a moisturizer during the day.

Remember, benzoyl peroxide is a bleaching agent, so if you are using it on your chest or back be careful about what you're wearing. Many a favourite T-shirt has been ruined!

ANTIBACTERIAL PREPARATIONS

Two other popular treatments for acne that can be bought at the pharmacist are Clearacil® and Valderma® preparations. These contain antibacterial agents that can kill the bacteria that cause acne.

Clearacil® contains 8 per cent sulphur and 0.1 per cent

triclosan. Valderma® contains 0.2 per cent chlorocresol and 0.2 per cent potassium hydroxyquinoline.

What Is It?
The antibacterial agents triclosan, chlorocresol and potassium hydroxyquinoline kill a wide range of bacteria including *Propionibacterium acnes*. The agents penetrate into the hair canal and kill the bacteria, thus preventing the inflammatory response. They have no effect on microcomedones, blackheads or whiteheads.

Sulphur has been used for decades in the treatment of acne. It has an effect on moulds and bacteria in the skin, but its exact mode of action is unclear.

How Long Does It Take to Work?
The effects of these agents can be fairly rapid to begin with, but the effects tend to slow down with use. If you have not achieved at least 50 per cent improvement in the first two months you are on the wrong treatment and should consult your doctor for further options.

Are There Any Side-effects?
These agents can cause some dryness of the skin. The use of a light moisturizer will help to settle this.

What Can I Get from My Doctor?

Benzoyl peroxide preparations can be prescribed by your doctor, and this may be the first treatment he or she gives you for your acne. If benzoyl peroxide does not work after a two-month period, you should be changed to a different type of treatment which should be an antibiotic solution, lotion or gel.

TOPICAL ANTIBIOTICS

Topical antibiotics have the advantage of achieving high concentrations at skin level, where they are needed, and avoiding the side-effects encountered when antibiotics are taken in tablet form (*see Chapter 5*). There are eight different antibiotic preparations available in the UK, which are described in the table below.

These preparations should be used twice daily over the whole area affected, not just to individual spots. They can be combined with a topical vitamin A preparation, using the vitamin A at night and the antibiotic during the day; they can also be used with a salicylic acid wash such as Acnisal® wash. All the antibiotic preparations have been shown to work, but there is a lot of individual variation as to which some people can tolerate and which ones work most quickly and well.

How Does It Work?

Antibiotic preparations work by penetrating into the skin and killing the *Propionibacterium acnes* which cause the inflammatory spots of acne. They have little effect in the non-inflammatory spots of acne, though the alcohol bases can help to unseat obvious blackheads. The exception to this is Isotrexin®, which combines the topical antibiotic with vitamin A and thus targets both inflammatory and non-inflammatory lesions.

With most topical antibiotics it is best to combine them with a vitamin A preparation which will clear the microcomedones and prevent new spots from coming up.

Topical Antibiotics

Trade Name	Constituents	Form
Topicycline®	0.22 per cent Tetracycline	Alcoholic solution
Stiemycin®	2 per cent Erythromycin	Alcoholic solution (not available in the US)
Dalacin T solution®	1 per cent Clindamycin	Alcoholic solution (marketed as Cleocin-T in the US)
Dalacin T lotion®	1 per cent Clindamycin	Creamy lotion
Zineryt®	4 per cent Erythromycin & 1.2 per cent zinc acetate	Alcoholic solution (not available in the US)
Benzamycin® gel	3 per cent Erythromycin & 5 per cent Benzoyl peroxide	White gel
Actinac®	1 per cent Chloramphenicol, 1 per cent hydrocortisone & 8 per cent sulphur	Lotion
Isotrexin® gel	2 per cent Erythromycin & 0.05 per cent Isotretinoin	Gel

Trade Name	Constituents	Form
Erygel	2 per cent Erythromycin	Gel (available in US only)

How Long Does It Take to Work?

With antibiotic skin preparations, I expect at least a 50 per cent improvement in the first two months of use. After this, the spots should clear in four to six months, though you may need to use the preparation whenever you feel a spot coming up. If you have not achieved this sort of response, the preparation is unlikely to totally clear the spots and you should be put on something stronger.

In general, best results are seen with Zineryt® and Benzamycin®, both of which work very rapidly. If you have been given Topicycline®, Stiemycin® or Dalacin T® and your acne has not cleared, it would be worth trying Zineryt® or Benzamycin®. Benzamycin®, perhaps (depending on how the individual responds and how well he or she tolerates the treatment), has the advantage of containing two active antibacterials which work together – both Erythromycin and benzoyl peroxide killing the bacteria.

Are There Any Side-effects?

The alcoholic solutions can all irritate the skin; if you have sensitive skin you may not be able to tolerate these. Most people with acne have very greasy skins; the alcohol helps to dry the skin out a little and thus the solutions are generally well tolerated. In people who find the alcoholic solutions too irritating to their skin, Dalacin T® does come in a creamy lotion specially formulated for more sensitive skin. Moisturizers can be used if the skin becomes dry or scaly.

Topicycline® is a slightly yellowish solution which can mark clothing, so be careful how you apply it. It also fluoresces under ultraviolet light – which can be used to great effect at the disco but can also be very embarrassing if you are not aware of this property.

Benzamycin® gel and Isotrexin® gel contain irritant components – benzoyl peroxide in Benzamycin® and isotretinoin in Isotrexin®. The antibiotics in these preparations, however, have anti-inflammatory properties and reduce the irritation of the complete preparation.

Zineryt® lotion has a fairly short shelf-life; once the bottle is opened it should be replaced after six weeks. Benzamycin® has a shelf-life of three months once opened but must be kept in the fridge or the shelf-life is significantly reduced.

All the antibiotics used in these skin preparations are now showing development of resistance to the bacteria in the skin. This is described in more detail in the next chapter. Resistance to the antibiotic may result in the preparation failing to work or the spots reappearing while still on treatment. Both Zineryt® and Benzamycin® have addressed this problem by including agents – zinc acetate and benzoyl peroxide – which the bacteria cannot become resistant to. This means that these preparations are more likely to give long-term results without the acne becoming 'used to' them.

Other Topical Preparations Used in Acne

A number of other skin preparations are used in mild-to-moderate acne. These work in different ways and may be very successful in acne. Peoples' response to them is variable; the only way of finding out whether they suit you is to try them.

PAPULEX® CREAM – TOPICAL VITAMIN B₃.

Papulex® cream was launched in 1995. It is based on vitamin B_3 and seems to have a good effect on inflammatory acne but has little effect on non-inflammatory acne. In some patients it appears to produce a certain amount of dryness of the skin but other patients tolerate it very well. In the UK and US it is only available on prescription, so you must get this from your doctor.

SKINOREN® CREAM

Skinoren® cream is based on azelaic acid. Azelaic acid has an antibacterial effect and also removes the dead cells from the top layer of the skin which helps to unblock hair canals. It thus has an effect on both inflammatory and non-inflammatory lesions of acne. Another effect azelaic acid has is on pigmentation in the skin. In darker skins, acne spots can result in unsightly dark marks on the skin (*see Chapter 8*). Although these are not permanent, they can last a long time. Skinoren® may in some individuals help to reduce these marks more quickly.

SHARK'S BILE EXTRACT – ISOLUTROL

Shark's bile extract was initially used in Japan in the treatment of acne and was found to reduce oil production in the skin. The active constituent is called Isolutrol and has now been produced in the laboratory and can be used without depleting the shark population. In the UK it is available as Ketsugol® and Solution 28,® both of which can be obtained without a prescription.

The response to this has been very variable. Some patients find it reduces the oil production in the skin, while others find it has little if any effect.

5

Treatment of Acne – Drugs Taken by Mouth

Moderate-to-Severe Acne

Antibiotic Tablets

In patients with moderate to severe acne, or patients whose acne has failed to respond to skin preparations, the treatment of choice is antibiotic tablets. These are only available on prescription in both the UK and US, so go and see your doctor. A number of these have proved to be very valuable in the treatment of acne, but the three most important things to remember when taking antibiotics are:

1 Take them correctly.
2 Take them for sufficient time.
3 Never stop them suddenly.

As a general rule, antibiotics should be taken at full dosage until the spots are clear, and should then be slowly reduced over a period of three to four months, to be replaced with an antibiotic skin preparation which will keep the skin clear. Studies have shown that the relapse rate is much lower if high doses of the antibiotic are given to begin with. Antibiotics should also be used with an agent that will unblock the hair canals and thus clear microcomedones and prevent new spots from developing. I usually offer patients vitamin A and a salicylic acid wash in conjunction with antibiotic tablets.

TYPES OF ANTIBIOTICS

We tend to classify antibiotics into first-line drugs, which we start with, and second-line drugs used if the first-line drugs fail to work or if the patient cannot tolerate them.

First-line antibiotics are tetracycline, oxytetracycline, erythromycin, lymecycline, vibromycin and minocycline. Second-line antibiotics include trimethoprim and clindamycin. The full doses and regimes for use are given in the table below.

The most commonly used antibiotics in acne are the tetracyclines. This is quite a large group of antibiotics which include tetracycline, oxytetracycline, minocycline, doxycycline and lymecycline. The older ones are oxytetracycline and tetracycline, and as these are the cheapest, they are often the first to be used by your doctor. The newer tetracyclines do have significant advantages over the older ones, however, and if the older ones fail to control your spots, drugs such as minocycline, doxycycline or lymecycline may be effective.

Antibiotic Tablets Used in Acne

Generic Name of Antibiotic	Full Dosage	Regime
oxytetracycline	1 g	250 mg four times daily
tetracycline	1 g	250 mg four times daily
erythromycin	1 g	250 mg four times daily
minocycline	100 mg	100 mg once daily
doxycycline	100 mg	100 mg once daily
lymecycline	408 to 816 mg	408 mg once or twice daily
trimethoprim	400 mg	200 mg twice daily
clindamycin	300 mg	150 mg twice daily

How Do I Take Antibiotics Correctly?

It is important that the amount of the antibiotic in the blood remains at a reasonably constant level. Certain drugs are taken into the bloodstream very quickly and disappear very quickly, therefore with these drugs you really have to take them four times a day to achieve good blood levels. Antibiotics that require four-times-a-day dosage include oxytetracycline, tetracycline and erythromycin. These antibiotics are also affected by food, particularly fats and carbohydrates, in the stomach – so if you have eaten before or within one hour of taking the tablet up to 70 per cent of the antibiotic is not absorbed and is thus wasted. If you are given one of these antibiotics you should take them on an empty stomach with water and not eat for one hour after. This is difficult, but the best results are seen if you take the tablets properly.

Trimethoprim and clindamycin have longer half-lives and can be taken twice daily. They are not affected by food and can be taken with meals.

The easiest antibiotics to take are minocycline, lymecycline and doxycycline, which have very long half-lives and can be taken once daily. They can also be taken with food, which means that compliance in taking the tablets is highest with these antibiotics.

Always remember that the major cause of failure of antibiotics to work is because they are not taken correctly.

How Do Antibiotics Work?

Antibiotic tablets work in acne by being absorbed into the blood and then into the skin where they kill the bacteria that cause the inflammatory spots of acne. As they go through the blood, they do not have a selective effect on the skin but can affect the whole body, which can lead to side-effects – see page 52. Antibiotics are specifically taken up in the oil gland and then into the hair canal where the bacteria reside. This can cause problems if your oil production is very high: If you have very oily skin, the antibiotic may be too diluted (by the oil in the skin) to work properly, and thus will not kill the bacteria. This is one reason for failure of antibiotics to work properly.

As well as having an antibacterial action, antibiotics also have an independent anti-inflammatory effect which helps to reduce inflammatory spots even quicker. Antibiotics have no effect on the non-inflammatory spots of acne; this is why they should always be used in conjunction with a vitamin A or salicylic acid preparation.

How Long Do They Take to Work?

When starting on antibiotic tablets always expect to be on them for at least six months, and probably longer. A course that is shorter than this is probably inadequate.

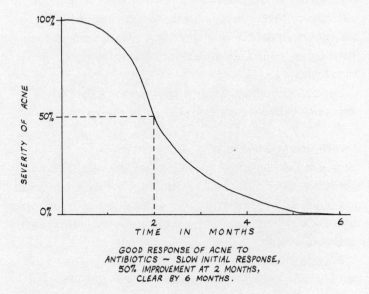

GOOD RESPONSE OF ACNE TO
ANTIBIOTICS — SLOW INITIAL RESPONSE,
50% IMPROVEMENT AT 2 MONTHS,
CLEAR BY 6 MONTHS.

Figure 12

If the antibiotics you are taking are going to be successful, you should expect a 50 per cent improvement in the first two months of treatment (Figure 12). Thereafter, the improvement continues and you should expect to be clear of new spots in four to six months. If you are not achieving this sort of progress, you are on the wrong treatment and it needs to be modified or changed.

Once you are clear of spots, the antibiotics should then be slowly tailed down. If taking oxytetracycline, tetracycline or erythromycin, these should be reduced by 250 mg per day each month – that is, initially you should be taking one tablet four times a day, then reduce this to three tablets per day for a month, then down to two a day for a month, then one a day for a month and then stop them. If the spots recur at any stage, go to the previous dosage until the skin is clear again and then try to reduce again. If on minocycline or doxycycline, reduce by 50 mg on alternate days each month (that is, day 1: 100 mg/day 2: 50 mg/day 3: 100 mg/day 4: 50 mg, etc.).

Never stop antibiotics suddenly. If you do the spots will come back with a vengeance.

Are There Any Side-effects?
All tablets have potential side-effects, and this is certainly true of antibiotics. The vast majority of side-effects seen with antibiotics are minor and are a nuisance at most. This is why most doctors do not hesitate in using antibiotic tablets in the treatment of acne.

Remember that when taking antibiotic tablets, they will not only affect the skin where you need the effect, but will also affect all parts of the body. This will alter the normal bacteria present in various sites of the body and this could cause symptoms. In women, this is very common in the vagina and allows the overgrowth of the yeast *Candida albicans*, with the resulting development of thrush. This is easily treated and tends not to recur. In the bowel, the change in the bacteria can cause minor symptoms such as nausea and mild diarrhoea, but this is self-limiting and usually only lasts for a few days. In some people there are no symptoms, but the change in the bacteria can affect the efficacy of the contraceptive pill if you are taking it (*see page 56*).

In occasional patients, vaginal thrush can be a recurring problem and the nausea can be persistent. In such patients it is worth trying to change the antibiotic, as they do not all have the same side-effects.

None of the antibiotics is totally safe in pregnancy; if you are a woman trying to start a family my advice would be to use only a topical treatment (*see Chapter 4*). The only antibiotic used in acne which can be used in pregnancy is erythromycin, but I would be very unhappy about a pregnant woman being on erythromycin for a long period of time.

Antibiotics can be associated with allergic skin rashes. These usually start seven to ten days after starting the antibiotic, covering the trunk and limbs with a red, bumpy and very itchy rash. This subsides after a week or so if the antibiotic is stopped. This is rare in the antibiotics used in acne, and is most common with trimethoprim.

Tetracyclines

Tetracyclines can cause brown discolouration of the teeth, and none of these – oxytetracycline, tetracycline, minocycline, doxycycline and lymecycline – should be used before the age of 13 when the teeth are still developing. After this age, they are safe and will have no effects on the teeth. In children under the age of 13, erythromycin tends to be used as it is safe and will not affect the teeth.

The tetracyclines can all make the skin more sensitive to the sun. In most people this means that they develop a darker and quicker tan. In some, however, the skin can become red, sore and itchy in sites exposed to the sun. The worst offender with this is doxycycline (Vibramycin®).

All the tetracyclines can also, very rarely, cause a slight increase in pressure around the brain, leading to persistent headaches. This condition is called benign intracranial hypertension. This is not dangerous and, if the tablets are stopped, it subsides very quickly. If you have persistent headaches, however, see your doctor.

The tetracyclines can also cause a form of arthritis. This is extremely rare and I have not seen a case of this in 15 years of treating acne sufferers with tetracyclines. The arthritis affects the hands, the feet, then the knees, hips and back. It can be associated with a general feeling of being unwell and there may be associated fevers and night sweats. This all clears when the antibiotic is stopped. Very bad acne can cause a form of arthritis by itself, so it may not be the antibiotics that are to blame and you should talk to your doctor about it.

There has been a lot of recent publicity about arthritis occurring with minocycline. The main problem with the reported cases was that the association of arthritis with minocycline was not recognized by the doctors looking after the patients and the patients suffered for long periods of time. It is important to remember that arthritis can be induced by any of the tetracyclines, is very rare and will get better if you stop the tetracycline. Use the tablets but be aware of the possible side-effects.

Erythromycin and the tetracyclines can cause an inflammation of the liver – a hepatitis. This is very rare and if the drug is stopped the hepatitis clears. There are a large number of commonly used drugs that can cause a hepatitis, mainly because the liver is the main site that drugs are broken down ready to be shed from the body. Hepatitis causes you to feel generally unwell and very intolerant of fat or alcohol, which make you nauseous. If you develop these symptoms see your doctor urgently.

In early 1995 there was a lot of press coverage about the potential side-effects of minocycline. This was very sensational and scare-mongering and caused real problems for many acne sufferers. Minocycline is an extremely valuable drug in that it is well-tolerated by the vast majority of patients and it shows very little in the way of drug resistance in the skin bacteria.

It has helped countless thousands of patients and still remains one of the most effective treatments for acne. As with all antibiotics it can cause problems, but these tend to be quite rare. Specific problems that can be seen with minocycline and not by the other tetracyclines are listed below:

1 **Skin pigmentation.** This tends to be a slate-grey pigmentation occurring in scarred areas. It can occur on any part of the body; if the drug is stopped when this first develops, it is reversible.
2 **Lupus-like syndrome.** Lupus erythematosus is a disease that can affect different parts of the body. Although its cause is unknown in most patients, certain drugs can induce a syndrome which mimics lupus erythematosus. Minocycline is one such drug, but this side-effect is very rare. It usually manifests as progressive arthritis affecting the hands, knees, hips and back, inflammation of the liver and a general feeling of malaise. This syndrome resolves when the drug is stopped.
3 **Allergic pneumonia.** This is very rare and presents with increasing breathlessness. It resolves when the drug is stopped.

These side-effects are rare and your doctor should be aware of the possibility that they can occur. Most of the problems encountered by patients who developed the lupus-like syndrome with minocycline were due to the fact that the drug was not recognized as the cause of the symptoms and was continued. Once the drug was stopped the symptoms resolved.

Antibiotics, as with any drugs, can have unusual side-effects in some people. Even simple drugs such as aspirin and paracetamol can have serious side-effects in some people. If you develop any symptoms that you cannot put down to a cough, cold or hay fever, do consult your doctor and specifically ask if the drugs you are on could be causing them.

ANTIBIOTICS AND THE CONTRACEPTIVE PILL

When you take the oral contraceptive the female hormones are absorbed into the bloodstream but are then taken up in the liver, combined with certain chemicals which inactivate them and then pass into the bowel in the bile. In the bowel, bacteria break down the hormone complex, activating the hormones which are then absorbed back into the bloodstream. This re-activation of the hormones is important for the efficacy of the Pill. Antibiotics can affect the efficacy of the contraceptive pill because the antibiotic kills bacteria in the bowel so that the hormones are not re-activated, which can make the Pill unsafe. The bacteria repopulate the bowel, even if antibiotics are continued, after 15 to 20 days; the Pill then becomes fully effective again.

If you are starting an antibiotic tablet for acne and are already on the contraceptive pill, it is important to use additional precautions, such as condoms, for the first month. If you are on an antibiotic for acne and then start the contraceptive pill, no additional precautions need to be taken except for those given when normally starting the Pill.

ANTIBIOTIC RESISTANCE

Bacteria are very primitive organisms but have an enormous capacity to survive. If they are exposed to an antibiotic for a period of time, they will change their genetic make-up to develop ways of avoiding the lethal effects of the antibiotics. This is happening in acne. The main bacterium involved in acne, *Propionibacterium acnes*, has developed more and more resistance to the antibiotics used in acne, over the years. In the 1970s, bacterial resistance was about 20 per cent to any of the antibiotics used in acne. It is now running at 70 per cent in specialist centres such as Leeds Royal Infirmary. Some of this resistance, or protection against antibiotics, is fairly low-level and the concentrations of antibiotics used in skin preparations or achieved in the skin with antibiotic tablets will still kill the bacteria. In those showing high-level resistance, the antibiotic will not work and this may be a reason for treatment failure. High resistance is now seen to erythromycin, oxytetracycline, tetracycline and clindamycin. Resistance is also now occurring to doxycycline and trimethoprim. The only antibiotic that there is still very low resistance to is minocycline.

In all patients being treated with antibiotics for acne, an agent that will kill bacteria but to which there is no resistance should be used periodically – that is, once a week or every two weeks. One agent that is usually recommended is benzoyl peroxide. The topical preparation Benzamycin® contains benzoyl peroxide and erythromycin, and thus fully addresses this problem of resistance.

CAN LONG-TERM ANTIBIOTICS HARM MY HEALTH?

There is a myth that antibiotics will affect your immunity and make you more prone to infections. There is no scientific evidence to support this. Unless you are developing side-effects from the antibiotic, they will not adversely affect your health even when used for years at a time. Within days of stopping the antibiotic, your body will have no memory that you have ever taken it.

Do remember that all tablets you take can have side-effects, and even if they are rare, they could affect you. If you develop any strange symptoms while taking antibiotics, do report them to your doctor.

Anti-inflammatory Drugs in Acne

Acne involves inflammation in the skin. The anti-inflammatory effect of antibiotics is part of the way that antibiotics work in acne. One other anti-inflammatory drug can have a powerful effect in acne: dapsone. This is not an antibiotic and its main use world-wide is in the treatment of leprosy. It has a powerful effect on inflammation in the skin and is used in a variety of inflammatory skin diseases where it reduces the migration of white blood cells into the areas of inflammation. In acne, dapsone was used extensively before the more widespread use of antibiotics, but is still very useful in combination with antibiotics. Used at a dose of 50 mg daily, dapsone will often convert a partial response to a complete response.

At high dosage, dapsone can cause thinning of the blood, inflammation of the liver, and skin rashes. In some people a deficiency of the enzyme glucose-6-phosphate dehydrogenase makes them more susceptible to the side-effects of dapsone, and catastrophic breakdown of red blood cells can occur. Anyone suspected of having this defect – that is, those of Afro-Caribbean or Mediterranean origin – needs to be specifically tested for this enzyme defect before the drug is given. At the small dose used in acne, dapsone is generally a

safe drug but the blood should be monitored if it is continued
for longer than three months.

Hormone Treatment

As detailed in Chapter 1, acne is caused by an increased
sensitivity of the skin to the male hormone, testosterone. In
women with acne, specific hormone treatment can be given
that will reduce the effect of the male hormone on the skin,
though this will have an effect on all parts of the body. This
cannot be used in men as it would essentially chemically
castrate them.

DIANETTE®

This is a combined hormone pill which contains a low level of
the female hormone oestrogen with a drug called cyproterone
acetate which counteracts testosterone. As well as being a
treatment for acne it is also a reliable contraceptive pill. As it is
not primarily sold in the UK as a contraceptive it cannot be
obtained from a Family Planning Clinic but has to be obtained
on prescription from your doctor.

How Does It Work?
The cyproterone acetate blocks the action of testosterone on
the skin and will, therefore, reduce oil production in the skin,
reduce microcomedone formation and thus suppress acne.

How Long Does It Take to Work?
In the first month of taking Dianette® there may be a slight
increase of spots. Thereafter the spots should subside and the
skin should be clear in four months. If the skin is not clear in

this time frame, it will probably not clear and additional or alternative treatment should be started. Dianette® can be safely used for many months and I have seen women who have used Dianette® for three or four years without problem. When the Dianette® is stopped the acne may flare up again, as there is no way of slowly reducing the dosage.

Are There Any Side-effects?

As with any contraceptive pill, Dianette® can cause mood swings. I have treated a number of women who became clinically depressed while taking Dianette®. Patients can experience weight gain and, in older women or women with risk factors such as high blood pressure and obesity, there is a risk of venous thrombosis.

OTHER HORMONE TREATMENTS

One other drug which has the effect of reducing the effect of testosterone on the skin can be used in women with acne. This is a drug called spironolactone. This drug is principally used as a diuretic (that is, a drug that makes you pass more urine). At low doses the diuretic effect is small, and its anti-male hormone effect can be a useful addition to antibiotics in women with acne. I use this drug at the dose of 50 to 100 mg daily. In women who experience a pre-menstrual exacerbation of their acne, spironolactone can be used for the seven days before the period and can be successful in reducing this flare-up. It can cause a mild increase in urine output, so I usually recommend that it is taken in the morning to avoid having to get out of bed at night to go to the toilet. In some women it can cause problems with their periods, with an alteration of the cycle, heavy bleeding or loss of periods. This comes back to normal when the drug is stopped.

Treatment for Severe Acne: Roaccutane®

In severe nodular cystic acne or acne that is not responding fully to long courses of antibiotics, the treatment of choice is the synthetic vitamin A derivative, Roaccutane® (generic name: isotretinoin). This is a very significant drug and the majority of patients treated with it will clear their acne completely in a four-month period. Some patients may need longer courses; I have treated one patient for nine months with Roaccutane®. About 50 per cent of patients are free of their acne thereafter, but the rest do relapse within the next year or two. The acne may come back in a minor way and be controlled with creams, or may come back severely and require further courses of Roaccutane®. There is no way of predicting this before you take the drug.

Although effective in most patients who are prescribed it, some patients are not able to tolerate it (*see page 66*), and in some patients it does not work. There is no way of telling if you are a non-responder before you take the drug.

In the UK, Roaccutane® is a drug that can only be prescribed by a dermatologist, so to get this drug you need to be referred to the hospital or must see a dermatologist privately. The dose of the drug is dependant on your body weight, the usual dose being 1 mg per kilogram body weight per day.

How Does It Work?
Roaccutane® is absorbed through the stomach and affects all parts of the body. The major effects are on the skin, where Roaccutane®:

1 reduces oil or sebum production by up to 90 per cent
2 changes the growth of skin cells in the hair canal, which

removes microcomedones and prevents them from
reforming
3 reduces inflammation in the skin
4 has an antibacterial effect.

In these ways, Roaccutane® stops all the changes in the skin
that cause acne, and the skin clears. When the drug is stopped,
oil production slowly recovers to normal levels within one
year, though in most patients microcomedones do not reform.

How Long Does It Take to Work?
In the first month on Roaccutane®, acne can become worse
rather than better. If you have particularly inflammatory acne,
it can become very much worse in the first month and your
dermatologist may put you onto a short course of systemic
steroids to prevent this from happening. In most patients,
acne slowly reduces in the first two months but there is then a
more rapid response and, again in most patients, the acne
clears completely in four months. Occasionally, patients do
require longer courses of Roaccutane® to achieve complete
clearance of the skin; the drug should be continued until all
the spots have subsided, which can take up to nine months.

Are There Any Side-effects?
The side-effects of Roaccutane® are generally related to its effect
on the sebaceous gland and oil production. The most common
side-effect is drying and chapping of the lips. Nearly everyone
put on the drug will experience this. Drying of the skin in
general is the next most common side-effect. If this becomes
severe, the skin can become very itchy. The hair becomes drier
and may need washing only once a week rather than every day.
The hair can, however, become brittle and may break, leading to

some hair loss. More rarely, the lining inside the nose can be affected, giving rise to soreness and nose bleeds. The eyes can also be affected, leading to grittiness of the eyes and problems with contact lenses if these are used. A similar effect in joints and muscles can lead to joint pain and muscle ache, particularly when exercising. A professional footballer I was treating had to stop Roaccutane® because the joint and muscle pain prevented him from training.

Roaccutane® can have an effect on the liver and may induce inflammation of the liver or hepatitis. This is why blood tests are performed before you are started on the drug. This side-effect is rare, and if the initial blood test is OK there is usually no problem.

Roaccutane® can also have an effect on the amount of fat in the blood. Your dermatologist will arrange a special blood test to be taken after you have been fasting overnight, to see how much fat is present in your blood. If you have a high level of fat you may need to be put on a low-fat diet when you are started on the drug.

As with most drug-induced side-effects, the above side-effects settle fairly quickly after the drug is stopped. Lots of lip salve and moisturizers are usually all that are needed. If drying in the nose is a problem, Vaseline® applied with a cotton bud and massaged into the nose can help. If the eyes become very gritty, artificial tears can be prescribed by your doctor to alleviate this.

Roaccutane® will damage unborn babies and it is very important that women do not become pregnant while they are on the drug. As it is retained in the fat for up to one month, adequate contraception must be continued for one month after stopping the drug.

There has been a lot of recent publicity about the effects Roaccutane® can have on the psychological well-being of people taking it. In one newspaper story, Roaccutane® was claimed to be responsible for severe depression in one young man who eventually committed suicide. This is obviously a very distressing case, but thankfully such side-effects are rare. The knowledge that this is a rare side-effect obviously does nothing to help the parents of the tragic youth and our sympathies must be with them. If you or a relative of yours is put on Roaccutane®, be aware of the possibility of depression and, if it occurs, consult your dermatologist immediately and discuss it with him or her.

Roaccutane® can cause a number of rare side-effects; if you develop any unusual symptoms while taking the drug, do contact your doctor.

In 10 per cent of patients who have been treated with Roaccutane®, long-term skin side-effects can occur. These are usually very minor, with mild dryness of the skin or persistent grittiness of the eyes. Two patients I have seen have developed more severe dryness of the face, which has caused them real embarrassment and discomfort. I cannot be certain that the Roaccutane® was the cause of this persistent dryness, but the onset occurred after the drug was started.

WHAT IF ROACCUTANE® DOES NOT WORK OR THE ACNE COMES BACK WHEN THE TREATMENT IS STOPPED?

Ninety-eight per cent of patients will respond to Roaccutane®, but in some this could mean up to a nine-month course before the skin is clear and the drug can be stopped.

This means that 2 per cent of patients will not respond to Roaccutane® – some may not be able to tolerate the side-effects of the drug and be forced to stop, others simply do not respond or even get worse on treatment.

It must be very depressing for these patients as they have effectively tried the most potent treatment for acne – and it has not worked! Don't despair! We treated acne before Roaccutane® was discovered and we can still effectively treat those who do not respond. This may mean taking a cocktail of antibiotics and anti-inflammatory drugs, but we eventually get the acne under control.

What about those who respond to Roaccutane® but then relapse months or years later? If the relapse is bad, a further course of Roaccutane® is an option but, in my experience, if you relapse after one course of Roaccutane® you will tend to relapse after the second, third, fourth ... I have been referred patients who have had six courses of Roaccutane®, and have relapsed after every one.

In general I will not prescribe another course of Roaccutane® if a patient has relapsed after a course. There are other ways of treating acne and only in the very few patients who do not respond to other treatments will I consider Roaccutane® again.

6

Other Treatments That Can Help in Acne

Sunlight

The majority of patients with acne say that they get better when they go on a sunny holiday, and often come back completely clear. In general, dry sunshine is very good, as patients are exposed to the beneficial effects of the sunlight without the problems associated with high humidity. If the humidity is high the moisture is taken up into the hair canal and can swell up the partial blockage that has developed, giving rise to acute blockages and a severe flare-up of the acne (*see Chapter 7*). A major problem for American soldiers in the Vietnam War was not a tropical illness but a fulminant form of acne where lakes of pus developed under the skin and the patients were left prostrate.

If you are planning a holiday, choose somewhere dry like

Greece, Spain or Arizona. Avoid humid environments like the
Caribbean or Florida.

How Does It Work?

It is not the ultraviolet light (the part of sunlight that gives
you sunburn and a suntan) that is important in the treatment
of acne, it is longer wavelengths in the red and blue spectrum.
These light rays excite chemicals called porphyrins, present in
the bacteria which cause inflammation in acne. These
porphyrins then kill the bacteria. It is like having an extra dose
of antibiotics.

Unfortunately, acne often flares up when you get home –
just like stopping antibiotics suddenly.

Artificial Light Treatment

In the past, ultraviolet light was used in the treatment of acne.
High doses were given which resulted in burning of the skin,
which subsequently peeled off. This was painful treatment
which was not very successful and has thankfully now been
abandoned.

Sunbed treatments will do very little for your acne. The
immediate tan that you develop can help to hide marks left by
acne, but the wavelengths of light emitted by these sunbeds
will have little effect on your acne, and will increase your risk
of developing skin cancer later in life.

In our laboratory, we have been investigating the effect of
sunlight on acne and have developed a form of light therapy
which produces the wavelengths of light that will excite
porphyrins and will kill the bacteria causing the inflammation

in acne. Light tubes producing light at 440 and 660 nanometers are set into a small facial tanning unit. Treatment takes 15 minutes a day (the eyes are protected with goggles). Trials on these light boxes have shown that they are more effective than benzoyl peroxide in the treatment of mild acne. We hope that these light boxes will be commercially available in the near future.

Chemical Peeling

Chemical peels with alpha hydroxyacids have been shown to help in the treatment of acne. These peels are used to help scarring in acne, but can be used while the acne is still active and can help to control the acne as well. Alpha hydroxyacids are fruit acids including glycolic acid. Chemical peels are usually given by plastic surgeons.

Vitamins in Acne

As an adolescent I was always told that vitamin B was good for spots and I took Brewer's yeast on a regular basis without any effect. As long as you have a good balanced diet, you are taking in all the vitamins you need and any extra are just eliminated from the body through the urine. Acne is not due to a deficiency in any vitamins.

Alternative Remedies

Traditional Chinese Medicine

Chinese herbal medicine has been documented for more than 2,000 years, and practised for at least 4,000. Outside China, Traditional Chinese Medicine (TCM) is generally used by doctors who are also trained and qualified in Western medicine, so that both disciplines are considered when treating a patient.

Skin conditions, acne among them, have been consistently shown to be very receptive to this form of alternative treatment. The basic principle of TCM is to treat the whole person, within the environment he or she inhabits. Practitioners believe that the illness or condition reflects an imbalance in the body; the purpose of the prescribed herbal mixture is to treat the underlying cause of the condition as well as the symptoms.

Chi (pronounced *chee*) is the English way of saying the Chinese word for the human life-force or energy *Qi* and it is this that the treatment aims to affect.

A traditional Chinese herbal doctor will want a very detailed case history of each new patient, which ideally starts from a detailed form filled in by the patient in advance of the first consultation. Then, from the moment you walk into the consulting room, the doctor is noticing things about you which he or she is trained to know are relevant to your health. The doctor will look at your tongue, noting its colour, coating and texture, and check the pulses in each wrist. There are 12 pulses – six on each wrist – which relate to different parts of the body and its organs. These pulses reflect the different imbalances in the system which are causing the symptoms in a particular patient in a particular way.

When the diagnosis has been made, the doctor will prescribe a selection of about 8 to 12 different herbs from a range of around 160. These are then weighed out in the dispensary and have to be taken home, cooked like a soup and drunk like a 'tea', usually between 100–150ml twice a day. At the beginning of the course of treatment a patient will generally need a bag of 'tea' for each day; as the condition improves this will usually decrease so you need one bag every two days, and so on. Sometimes creams, lotions, washings, compresses and masks are also prescribed to be used on the skin.

At the start of treatment you drink your 'tea' twice a day. The universal opinion as far as the taste and smell of these concoctions is everything from disgusting to vile – although it is suggested that if you like liquorice it's not too bad – but patients who undertake a course of Chinese medicine soon find their own way of coping with this.

After a week or two, at your next visit, the doctor will assess the progress of the treatment. One of the advantages of the herbal prescriptions is that they are 'tailor-made' and very adaptable. The doctor can alter the herb mixture, adding a little more of this and giving a little less of that, or try different herbs completely – in an effort first to stabilize the condition and then to decrease its effect, with the ultimate aim of eliminating it completely. The permutations are almost endless and it means that prescriptions are finely tuned to suit each individual patient.

If circumstances change in the patient's life in some way during treatment – an added stress, like moving house, or perhaps a pleasant experience, like falling in love – or if the weather becomes much hotter or colder, for instance – these factors will be taken into consideration as the doctor monitors the patient's progress.

HOW DOES IT WORK?

Chinese medicine works from the inside out. Very often people with chronic skin conditions are able to understand this better than people with other medical problems. Acne sufferers, in particular, are used to taking something by mouth to treat their skin, as well as treating the skin itself, from the outside, so they are often more receptive to the concepts of Chinese herbal treatments.

However, if a patient has suffered acne for some years, has tried the usual sources of help with little success and is becoming desperate, it makes it more difficult for the Chinese doctor to prescribe a treatment which will work as quickly as the patient would like. Acne patients apparently have a reputation for being more impatient than others, and some give up and go away after a six-week course. But others are more persevering.

At the same time, a skin condition sufferer may have learned enough to know that hoping for a complete 'cure' is perhaps unrealistic. They may be able to understand that a gradual but impressive improvement in their skin is worth a great deal, and may persist for longer.

Those who are committed to TCM believe that the treatments can also be used as preventive medicine. Many patients find that after a course of treatment their condition stabilizes and they are able to stop. They use the prescription only as an occasional booster or reviver to keep things under control.

Case Histories

Charles tried TCM when he was 17. His acne was troubling him and he'd asked to see the family doctor about it. His mother was anxious about the prescription for antibiotics he'd been given, however, and suggested he try Chinese herbal medicine. She'd heard good reports of the treatment from a friend whose child had suffered from eczema. Charles says:

And it did work. It's all rather mysterious, with all the herbs, and it's a slow and gradual effect, but it calmed it down and 18 months later it's still under control. Mum made up the tea, which was horrible – I hate liquorice – and although the acne isn't completely cured, I can always go back and use the creams they prescribe or have more treatment. I'd rather go back to the Chinese doctors – they're all pretty friendly there.

Charles' mother told me she and her husband had asked Charles if his acne was bothering him and offered help, but she said they hadn't wanted to put pressure on him to do anything he didn't want to.

His face was very red and inflamed at the time, and it had been getting worse for the previous couple of years, but I didn't like the idea of the antibiotic treatment over a long period because I think you get immune to it. As a family, we've tried other alternative medicine before – homoeopathy, particularly – and I'd heard from a friend whose baby had very bad eczema that Chinese medicine could help with skin problems.

I made up the herbal tea and tasted it myself. It wasn't too bad, although Charles didn't like it much. But it seemed to work for him.

Louise has suffered from acne, on her face, back and chest, since she was 13 or 14. She's now 39.

Over the years I've tried every treatment under the sun. At the moment, it's the best it has ever been. I tried TCM because I'd reached a point of desperation. I hadn't really been to the doctor about it since my teens, but at the age of 30 I went back to my doctor because it had flared up again and I was fed up with it. He put me on antibiotics and I was on them for about two years. I also tried Retin A®, but that really burned my skin. Then my husband read an article about Chinese herbal medicine and how it could help skin conditions like eczema, and we made enquiries.

I was on the treatment for about five months in all. I drank the tea for three months. It smells pretty awful while you're cooking it and I can't imagine what the neighbours thought I was brewing up in my kitchen, but it doesn't taste too bad. Then I took the little tablets they prescribe for another two months and it seemed to be under control, so I stopped.

Since then I've had a baby. The acne flared up while I was pregnant, but I was advised against going back on the treatment during pregnancy. It's always worse in the winter and is definitely connected with my menstrual cycle. It's better than it has ever been, but I've now accepted the fact I'll never have perfect skin.

Acne has definitely affected my life, and it still stops me from doing lots of things. At school I tended to hide and keep quiet and I think now that it prevented me from taking the opportunity of going to university – because I could have done. My husband tells me that people don't notice it as much as I do, but I'm not convinced. I have a baby daughter and when she's older, there's no way I'll let her suffer with acne, as I did.

Pregnant women (and children under one year) cannot be treated with traditional Chinese medicine.

There are now many TCM health centres internationally. If you don't know anyone who can give you a personal recommendation, try the Yellow Pages. Don't be shy about shopping around until you find the Chinese herbal doctor you feel most comfortable with.

In the UK, the Chi Centre (*see Useful Addresses*) is affiliated to the Institute of Complementary Medicine. The Centre operates a Chi Helpline (0171-222 1888) so that anyone who wants to know about Chinese herbal medicine in general and find out whether it might help their particular condition can talk to someone who knows.

COSTS

Fees will vary from clinic to clinic. In London in 1998, the Chi Centre charged £70 for the first consultation, which includes the prescribed herbs for the first week. Thereafter, the 'tea' costs either £40 per week or £40 for two weeks, depending on your condition. Creams, lotions and the tablets sometimes used as a 'top-up' are a bit extra.

ASPECTS TO CONSIDER

As with any 'alternative' treatment there is always an element of sceptical opinion. Some Western doctors believe that successes have more to do with 'mysticism' than medicine, or believe that the condition would have improved or disappeared anyway. There have also been some cases of poisoning, apparently as a result of herbal treatments.

But if a patient feels better about him- or herself internally after the experience of being treated with traditional Chinese medicine, then he or she is likely to feel and look better externally – which in the case of skin conditions is the main purpose of treatment.

So use your personal judgement. Find out about TCM, check out the credentials of the clinic or doctor you are considering, and then keep an open mind about the success of the treatment for your particular condition.

Acupuncture

Acupuncture springs from the same traditional Eastern beliefs about healing the body, mind and spirit. Acupuncturists also work with the flow of the body's energy, the *Qi*, which travels beneath the surface of the skin through a network of invisible channels, or meridians. The aim is to restore the balance between the equal but opposing elements of this energy, known as the Yin and the Yang.

The acupuncturist's needles are inserted into acupuncture points in very specific locations along the 12 main meridians, which relate to the relevant organs of the body.

HOW DOES IT WORK?

As with other Eastern medical practitioners, the first consultation is very detailed and takes note both of what you say in response to questions about yourself and your lifestyle, and the way you say it.

During acupuncture treatment, tiny needles are inserted into the skin for a second or two, or left in place under careful supervision for up to 20 or 30 minutes. Sometimes a herbal preparation known as moxa is burned on or near the acupuncture point and removed when it feels hot. Similarly, a small electric current can also be used through the needles. The sensation when the sterilized needles are inserted is rarely described as painful. Most people feel a 'heaviness' of the limbs, or a mild tingling, along with a pleasant feeling of relaxation.

Lasers are nowadays sometimes used on the acupressure points, especially for those with a phobic fear of needles.

Treatment can be very swift, or can last for several months. The British Acupuncture Council says, 'there is usually some change after about five treatments.'

Case History

Alison says of her acupuncturist:

He was wonderful. If pure faith could have cured me, I think he would have. I really felt we were a team. He took time with me and made me feel as if I was being considered not just as a person with spots – he was looking at the whole picture. He tried really hard.

HOW TO FIND A REGISTERED ACUPUNCTURIST

In Britain, many acupuncturists are also medical doctors or qualified physiotherapists, and more and more patients are being referred for treatment by their doctors. In 1995 the British Acupuncture Council (*see Useful Addresses*) was formed as a development of the former Council for Acupuncture, as a governing body for the growing profession to set and maintain standards and provide a referral system to accredited practitioners, through the Register of Practitioner Members. Members have the letters MBAcC after their name.

There are similar standardizing bodies for complementary medicine in the US, Canada and Australia. Please consult your doctor, local library or Yellow Pages.

Homoeopathy

This is probably the most accepted and well-established form of complementary or alternative medicine available in the UK. Its principles were discovered and developed by Dr Samuel Hahnemann during the 19th century and, since 1948, patients have been referred for treatment by doctors, either at one of five NHS Homoeopathic hospitals, or privately. Many practitioners are conventionally medically trained and registered with the Faculty of Homoeopathy (*see Useful Addresses*), but others come from a non-medical background and are registered as members of the Society of Homoeopaths.

ABOUT HOMOEOPATHY

The basic principles include the practice of treating 'like with like', and that a substance which might cause symptoms in a well person will cure similar symptoms in an unwell person. Practitioners also work on the basis of prescribing the smallest possible amount of a remedy in the belief that the more it is diluted, the more potent its effect.

Remedies are matched to the 'whole' person and accurate prescribing is considered to be the test of a good homoeopath. There are more than 2,000 homoeopathic remedies, all made from products found in nature.

Treatment is in the form of tiny tablets, powder, granules or liquids, all taken by mouth.

HOW DOES HOMOEOPATHY WORK?

Homoeopaths consider that symptoms of illness are the body's way of showing that the 'normal' self-healing system is not working well enough or is failing. The prescribed remedy is intended to match the symptoms on the basis of the homoeopathic belief that two comparable illnesses cannot exist in the body at the same time. By adding a harmless clone of the illness, the existing disease can be eliminated, after which the 'clone' disappears. The principles of treatment are aimed at stimulating the body's own defence mechanisms and ability to control the disease.

DOES IT WORK FOR ACNE?

It seems a great many acne sufferers have tried homoeopathic treatments, but none could be found who claimed an impressive effect.

Some people found more sympathetic understanding from a homoeopathic doctor, but found the treatments worked very slowly.

The reference to the causes for acne in *Homoeopathic Medicine – a Doctor's Guide to Remedies for Common Ailments* by Trevor Smith, referred to by the Faculty of Homoeopathy, is far from encouraging: 'Causes – Diet over-rich in carbohydrates, constitutional, lack of hygiene'.

Having said this, self-help homoeopathic treatments are available from large national pharmacists and health food shops. Sulphur, hepar sulph, pulsatilla and silicea seem to be recommended.

7

What Makes Acne Worse?

Acne is a very distressing condition mainly because it is so visible. Society tells us the whole time that we need to have perfect skin, and when a blemish develops on the skin nobody likes it! It does get to the point with a lot of my patients that they cannot bear to look at themselves in the mirror, and many patients take down all mirrors in their home so they can't look at themselves at all. Indeed, one patient would lie in bed and feel her face to see how many spots had come up overnight before even getting out of bed.

Obviously the best way of getting over all of this is by getting the acne clear, and that demands good, active treatment. This is as much to do with you as with your doctor or dermatologist. They can always prescribe treatments but it is you that has to use them – and use them properly! It is, therefore, very important to understand what the treatment is, how it works and how to use it correctly. Also you need to know what possible side-effects there are so that you can identify them, and what you should expect from the treatment.

As you will see from Chapters 3, 4, 5 and 6, all treatments should give at least 50 per cent response in the first two months of therapy. If you're not achieving this then you're on the wrong treatment!

I very much believe in a holistic approach to the treatment of any disease. You cannot take a person as purely their skin without looking at the rest of the body and how it interacts with the skin. Having a good, healthy lifestyle, therefore, increases your chance of getting a good response to the therapy.

Things That Will Exacerbate Acne

As you will see from Chapter 2, there are large numbers of myths surrounding what causes acne and what will make it worse. The vast majority of these are incorrect and can be totally disregarded. There are, however, a number of things that *can* make acne worse. If you are aware of these then they can be avoided. Forewarned is forearmed.

Things that we know will increase acne are listed below. Some we can control or at least modify, others we cannot.

1 stress, either at work or at home
2 hormones
3 sweating and high humidity
4 temperature
5 generally poor diet

6 occupation

7 picking and squeezing at the skin

8 drugs taken for other medical conditions

9 cosmetics.

1 Stress

Stress will exacerbate any skin condition, including psoriasis and eczema as well as acne. The mechanism by which this occurs is unknown, but it is very common. I have looked after four women who have cancelled their weddings on at least one occasion. Each time they neared their wedding day, stress levels increased and their spots became so bad that they cancelled because they could not bear the thought of wedding photographs of themselves covered with spots. I have now succeeded in getting all four women married – so there is always hope!

There have been some scientific studies that have shown a direct correlation between a flare-up of inflammatory acne and a very stressful and anger-inducing interview. A lot of my own patients invariably see a flare-up of acne before school exams or university exams, at the time of major stress such as losing their job or the break-up of a relationship, or even prior to a major event such as a wedding.

Our society is a stressful society. We all have stress at work, leisure and at home. Coping with stress certainly helps in controlling acne, and studies have shown that both psychotherapy and cognitive therapy help to improve the response of acne to conventional medical therapy.

Stress is something that few of us can do much about. The stress of exams, of a high-powered job, of deadlines is with us all and is very much a part of modern life.

The Acne Support Group has now commissioned relaxation tapes to help with stress, and specifically uses relaxation as a therapeutic aide in acne. These tapes first give a relaxation exercise which is almost like auto-hypnosis. It concentrates the mind on relaxation and allows you to dispel a lot of the stresses of daily life. The second side of the tape then shows you how you can specifically use relaxation to target the problems that you encounter with acne. These tapes are available from the Acne Support Group (*see Useful Addresses*).

2 Hormones
HORMONES IN WOMEN – POLYCYSTIC OVARY SYNDROME

As you will see from Chapter 1, acne, in general, is not caused by the presence of abnormally high hormones but is an over-reaction in the skin to normal hormone levels. Having said this, up to 50 per cent of women when tested do show a mild hormonal abnormality. In the vast majority of women this does not need to be treated and these women will respond to normal conventional treatment for their acne. The one exception to this is polycystic ovary syndrome.

In this syndrome multiple small cysts develop in the ovaries, and this is associated with higher levels of circulating male hormone. Blood tests will identify the elevated levels of free male hormone and ultrasound can identify the cysts within the ovaries.

Polycystic ovary syndrome can manifest itself in very different ways in different women. In some women it will cause menstrual irregularities, in others increased body hair (particularly in the beard area), in others acne and in still others, obesity. Polycystic ovary syndrome is a cause of infertility but it does not *always* cause infertility.

In women who have bad acne that is not responding well to treatment and have associated increased body hair or menstrual irregularities, I will usually send off a blood test for a hormone assay just to see whether they could have polycystic ovary syndrome.

One of the treatments of choice for polycystic ovary syndrome is Dianette®, which blocks the male hormone and helps acne, increased body hair and the menstrual disturbances.

The Contraceptive Pill

There are two types of oral contraceptives, the combined oral contraceptive – where two female hormones, oestrogen and progesterone, are present – and the progesterone-only contraceptive pill. In general, the hormone oestrogen counteracts the male hormone testosterone, and this will reduce the severity of acne. Progesterone, however, can be broken down in the liver to produce testosterone-like hormones which can make acne worse. It is very important, therefore, when using an oral contraceptive to avoid progesterone-only contraceptives, as these could make acne worse rather than better, and to make sure that you are given a combined oral contraceptive that is 'acne friendly' (that is, contains a progesterone that is not broken down into a male hormone-like hormone).

The commonest progesterones used in the oral contraceptive pill, levonorgestrel and norethisterone, can have marked male hormone side-effects which may exacerbate acne. These progesterones are present in a wide range of contraceptive pills sold in the UK, including (brand names) Loestrin®, Brevinor®, Microgynon®, Ovranette® and Eugynon®. The newer progesterones such as desogestrel, norgestimate and gestodene do not have this problem of being broken down into male hormone-like hormones. These progesterones are present in the oral contraceptive pills Marvelon®, Femodene® and Cilest®. If you have acne and want to start the oral contraceptive, do ask your doctor or Family Planning Clinic for an acne-friendly pill!

Pre-menstrual Exacerbation

It is very common for acne to flare up in the week or so prior to the period. This is because the hormone oestrogen, which normally counteracts the male hormone testosterone, falls rapidly coming up to the period. This effectively makes the male hormone more dominant and can lead to more spots developing. There are ways that this can be managed, which are outlined in Chapter 5.

HORMONES IN MEN

In men, hormone levels are never elevated in acne. The sebaceous glands do, however, have the capacity to respond to extra male hormone that is taken into the body. This is the reason that body-builders who use anabolic steroids often develop severe acne, particularly in the trunk. This can happen in men who have never had problems with acne before, as well as those who do have a problem with acne. To spend time, effort, energy and money to develop a body that you are proud of only to find that it is covered in spots and you are too embarrassed to show it must be very depressing. For all those would-be Chippendales: avoid anabolic steroids.

3 Sweating and High Humidity

As you will see from Chapter 1, the primary abnormality in acne that leads to the development of spots is the partial blockage in the hair canal, or microcomedone. When this partial blockage seals completely, oil builds up under the skin within the hair canal and this leads to an overgrowth of the bacteria and, eventually, inflammation. This partial blockage or microcomedone is composed of dead skin cells, and if these dead skin cells are rapidly hydrated they can swell and this can lead to an acute blockage of the canal and inflammatory spot formation.

This can happen when sweat is retained against the skin, particularly when tight-fitting underwear is used. It can also happen in very humid atmospheres. Problems can occur when acne sufferers go to very humid countries such as the Caribbean and some parts of South East Asia. If you want a sunny holiday abroad, go for the Mediterranean or south-western US; avoid the high humidity of the Caribbean.

Any activity that increases the humidity to which the skin is exposed can make acne worse. One patient whom I recently saw religiously took steam baths, feeling that the steam would open his pores and would help his acne. He did not realize until I pointed it out to him that invariably two or three days after going to the steam bath his acne would take a turn for the worse and he would develop many more inflamed spots. When he stopped his steam baths his acne improved rapidly. Avoid steam baths, avoid saunas and never use a facial sauna, as this could potentially make the spots worse and certainly no better.

4 Temperature

One of the primary changes in acne is an increase in the amount of oil produced in the skin. Oil production in the skin is mainly controlled by the male hormone, however, ambient temperature does have an effect and when the temperature rises so does the oil production. This is why most people tend to feel greasier in the summer when it is hot, and a lot of people find that their spots become worse in the summer. Although the heat in the summer is bad for your acne, sunshine is good for it, as sunshine has almost an antibiotic effect on the skin and will help to get rid of a lot of the bacteria that are causing the inflammatory spots. The cooler you can keep in the summer, the better your skin will tend to be.

5 Generally Poor Diet

As you will have read from Chapter 2, fried and fatty foods do not make acne worse. A generally poor diet will, however, have an impact on the whole body and may make acne worse. A good balanced diet is, therefore, important.

6 Occupation

Certain occupations can expose people to chemicals which can either cause acne or exacerbate pre-existing acne. One set of chemicals, the polycyclic aromatic hydrocarbons, cause a particular form of acne called chloracne. Occupational exposure to these chemicals may be seen in those handling or manufacturing dielectrics, insecticides, herbicides, fungicides and wood preservatives. The acne they develop is a very inflammatory form of acne which affects the face and trunk.

In workers working with cutting oils, acne-like eruptions can occur, particularly on the legs where oil soaks into overalls and other clothing and is retained against the skin. This is not true acne but more a folliculitis or inflammation of the hair follicle, aggravated by contact with the oil.

7 Picking and Squeezing at the Skin

As well as causing scarring, picking and squeezing your skin can cause more spots to come up. Part of this is due to swelling caused by squeezing the skin, which can cause acute occlusions of the hair canals by pressure on the upper part of the canal. This leads to oil accumulation and inflammation. Try to keep your hands away from your skin – you will only make it worse.

8 Drugs Taken for Other Medical Conditions

A number of medications used for a wide variety of conditions can cause or exacerbate acne. It is obviously important to be aware of this and, where possible, to get your doctor to prescribe alternatives that do not have this effect. The main medications that can cause or exacerbate acne are steroids, including corticosteroids, androgenic or male steroids, and anabolic steroids. As you can see from the section above on the contraceptive pill, the female hormone progesterone can also exacerbate acne.

Another major group of drugs that can cause severe acne are those used in epilepsy. Almost all the anti-epilepsy drugs can exacerbate acne, but some do so more than others. A few other drugs such as lithium (which is used to treat depression), isoniazid (used to treat tuberculosis) and iodides and bromides can also exacerbate acne.

9 Cosmetics

The vast majority of cosmetics now available are rigorously tested, usually on human volunteers, to see whether they will block pores and cause blackheads or comedones. A lot of products will carry the label 'non-comedogenic' or 'non-acnegenic', which means that they are friendly for use in people who have acne. It is not, however, just the cosmetics you might expect would cause problems, such as foundations and powders, that are the culprits. Blushers, lipsticks, eye shadows, moisturizers and sun-screens can also cause blackheads and other skin problems.

Always look at the labelling on your cosmetics before you buy them, to make sure that they are acne-friendly. Cosmetics which conceal spots are very important in the management of acne, acting as a much needed psychological prop for sufferers – both men and women. It is important, therefore, not to avoid the use of cosmetics but to make sure you choose the correct ones. In choosing your cosmetics always make sure that the product is non-comedogenic. Use low-oil or oil-free moisturizers.

8
❧

Management of Scarring

One of the major side-effects of acne is physical scarring of the skin. The different types of scarring are detailed in Chapter 1. Essentially, scarring in acne can be of two types: pitted and keloid.

Pitted Scarring

Pitted scarring generally results from more severe and deeper acne. Most of this is due to deep inflammation which causes destruction of the collagen, which supports the skin, and either allows the skin to dimple into the hole or else the scar attaches to the epidermis and pulls it down into sharp 'ice-pick' scars.

It is very important to remember that scarring is due to loss of substance in the skin. Many people will develop a mark where a spot has been. This may be red or, in darker skins, it can be very dark. The red marks represent blood vessels under the skin that have proliferated in response to the inflammation of the acne spot. Eventually the body remodels these blood vessels and the red mark resolves. The dark marks are what we call post-inflammatory pigmentation and are due to stimulation of the pigment-producing cells in the skin by the inflammation in the acne spot. The excess pigment gets lodged deep in the skin, in the dermis, and can persist for months or even years. Treatment does not really help these marks but a suntan can help to hide the dark marks. It is important to remember that these marks are not scars and will eventually settle with no treatment.

With pitted scarring, where the skin is dimpled, the scars may improve by themselves with time. As you will see from Chapter 4, vitamin A creams can help in this as they induce a new layer of collagen to be formed just under the skin. This acts as a pillow which pushes the skin out, smoothing out fine dimpled scarring. This does not happen quickly and you need to be patient with it.

Collagen Injections

One way of addressing soft pitted scars which gives immediate results is the use of collagen injections. In this technique, purified collagen is injected into the deeper layer of the skin or dermis and provides an immediate cushion which pushes the skin up and removes the defect that causes the scar. Initially the scar will look raised and lumpy, as excess collagen needs to be injected in. As the collagen settles everything levels out and the skin becomes flat again. The injections can be painful.

Results using collagen injections are good but are not permanent. The injections need to be repeated every six months to two years, as the collagen is slowly absorbed by the body and thus removed from the injection site.

Some people can have an allergic reaction to the injected collagen, so the doctor will initially put a small injection into your arm to see if you react to it. This he or she will examine three to seven days later and if there is no reaction will go ahead and give the collagen injections.

Always go to a recognized plastic surgeon or dermatological surgeon to have this done. Get advice from your doctor and get referred to someone he or she recommends. Some clinics try to inject scars which will not respond to this type of treatment, such as ice-pick scars, and can charge exorbitant prices.

Surgical Treatment of Scars

In deeper pitted scars where the scar margins are firm, there is more scar tissue present and these will tend not to improve with time and do not respond well to vitamin A creams. These scars require surgical intervention with chemical peeling, dermabrasion or laser resurfacing. All these techniques take off the top layer of the skin and with it some of the scar and then allow the skin to recover with an overall improvement in the skin's appearance.

DERMABRASION

In this technique, a small diamond burr is used to scrape the top layers off the skin. This is rather like having a deep graze. The skin recovers from bits of epidermis left and from hair canal skin cells and the improvement achieved can be up to 70 per cent. In people with very pale skin, the healed skin can be very red and can remain red for some time. In darker skins, the healed skin can become very dark and this may be permanent. Dermabrasion is, thus, not for everybody. If you have large deep scars, these can be individually removed by surgery to give flat line-like scars which can then be improved by dermabrasion later.

As you would expect, the skin takes some time to heal; expect to be out of circulation for three or four weeks after the procedure.

If you are thinking about dermabrasion, get your doctor to refer you to a plastic surgeon who can give you proper advice. Some UK plastic surgeons will provide dermabrasion on the NHS – this very much depends on where you live. Never answer ads in newspapers!

LASER RE-SURFACING

This technique is very new and there are only a few surgeons in the UK who have good expertise in it. Laser resurfacing uses CO_2 lasers to remove the top layers of the skin in much the same way as dermabrasion but everything is more finely tuned and the skin is not traumatized as much so the redness in pale skin and darkness in dark skin is less marked.

Laser resurfacing is generally not available on the NHS and can be very expensive. One of my patients was charged £4,000 to have his face laser re-surfaced in 1997. This was performed in a private clinic and I was hard pressed to see any difference in his skin after the procedure. Always be referred by your dermatologist to a good plastic or dermatological surgeon to get the best opinion and result.

CHEMICAL PEELING

In this technique a chemical – which could be phenol, trichlo-racetic acid or an alpha hydroxyacid – is applied to the skin to remove the top layer of the skin by 'burning it off'. It does the same sort of thing as dermabrasion but to a lesser extent. It is most suitable for finer scarring. The dead skin forms a mask which then peels off. The effects of chemical peeling continue over a six-month period, with deposition of new collagen deep in the skin so that the appearance of the skin continues to improve. Chemical peeling is generally not available on the NHS.

Keloid Scars

These are hypertrophic scars which can occur even after fairly trivial acne. They grow slowly and can reach 5 cm across. They are tender or itchy and very embarrassing. The best way to deal with these scars is to inject them with steroids. The injection must be given into the body of the scar and is painful. The injection stops the keloids from growing and eventually flattens them. The tenderness and itching are the first things to respond, after which the scar softens and flattens. Even when the keloid is flat you will always, however, be left with a cosmetic defect.

If keloids are surgically removed they invariably recur. Sometimes, very persistent ones can be surgically removed and the new scar treated with radiotherapy to prevent the keloid from reforming. This works in some people but has failed in two patients I have recently treated.

A novel approach is the use of cryotherapy or freezing therapy to treat keloids. In this, liquid nitrogen at minus

185°C/–301°F is sprayed onto the keloid. This destroys the cells that are forming the keloid. I have not had a lot of success with it but some groups have reported good responses. Laser treatment has also been used in keloids, but with more variable results.

Where to Get Treatment for Scarring

Keloids are generally treated by a dermatologist. Keloids may require multiple injections over a period of months or years to flatten them, so it demands patience from patient and doctor.

Dermabrasion, chemical peeling and laser re-surfacing are all provided by a plastic surgeon or dermatological surgeon. Always ask your doctor or dermatologist to refer you to someone they know is good and caring. Never answer newspaper advertisements or you will end up paying a lot of money and may not be happy with the end result.

ACNE SCARRING IS PREVENTABLE – PREVENTION IS BETTER THAN CURE. GET YOUR ACNE TREATED BEFORE SCARS DEVELOP.

9

Skin Care and Makeup Techniques

Making the Best of What You Have

Most of us dislike some part of our bodies – hate is too strong a word, although it's the one we'd probably use. We think our legs are too fat, or too thin, or too short – many women bemoan their pear-shaped figures or wish they had bigger, or smaller breasts. Men wish they were taller, or become obsessed with a hopeless ambition to prevent themselves becoming bald.

But unless we are in the depths of gloom, most of us could find something about ourselves which we like or we'd describe as OK. We may have big hips but we feel lucky to have thick, shiny hair which behaves well and is easy to style, for instance.

Faces are more specific and we have stronger feelings about them, perhaps because they mirror much more than anything else about us, our personality and the way we feel about ourselves. If we hate something about our face we can sometimes do something about changing it, like paying for a 'nose job' or having a face-lift.

If you have acne on your face, this book is about doing something about it – at the same time, you can also learn to make the most of what nature has given you by thinking and feeling good about looking good.

Even if you suffer from acne, we believe it's possible to make the most of yourself and look as good as you can. And the feeling that you've done your best gives you that little extra bit of confidence to go out into the world and face it!

But let's start at the beginning.

Facial Skin Care for Women

Cleansing and Cleansers

For people who have acne on their face, washing with soap and water is not ideal, even for those with very greasy skin. Facial cleansing bars, often described as 'pH balanced' and sometimes containing a moisturizer or antibacterial additives, are better. Facial wash lotions or gels are comparable and, being in plastic containers, are less messy and easier for travelling.

Astringents are good for those with oily skin, as they close the pores after cleansing and reduce the amount of sebum produced. Often these contain alcohol, which also removes any traces of the cleanser used. Apply an astringent before applying makeup, to reduce the risk of blackheads and help the makeup last longer.

Exfolients encourage the removal of dead skin cells, but those containing minute granules, such as crushed peach or avocado stones, should never be used on acne pustules.

For deeper cleansing, regular facials, such as mud packs, can be helpful on problem skin and these can be applied at home or at a beauty salon, by a qualified beauty therapist. Such treatment isn't recommended more than once a week.

BATH AND SHOWER PRODUCTS

As with facial cleansers, choose a pH-balanced, oil-free product. And although some products are sold as 'hair and body shampoos' it is better to use separate products on your hair and on your body.

SHAMPOOS AND CONDITIONERS

Often oily skin can be accompanied by greasy or lank hair. Hair that is totally degreased is dull, lifeless and brittle, so always choose a shampoo designed for your hair-type, for example for greasy/oily hair. A conditioner for your hair-type is also best, preferably the wash-in/wash-out type.

Most hairdressers recommend using separate shampoo and conditioner rather than the two-in-one varieties.

Moisturizers

Moisturizers retard the loss of natural moisture from the skin, preventing dryness and other cell damage. Choose a product which is described as 'oil free' and preferably also 'non-comedogenic', or 'non-acnegenic' (that is, less likely to give rise to blackheads) and always use it on a 'test area' to make sure it doesn't cause a reaction on your skin.

Moisturizers designed for use during the day, under make-up, leave the skin feeling silky and less 'tight'. They should be applied after using an astringent, and before applying a foundation.

However, some foundations contain enough moisturizer in themselves, and don't require a layer underneath. Do what feels best for your skin.

Foundations

These provide a base for the rest of your makeup. It's important to choose an appropriate shade for your skin type and colour.

Choose a foundation product which is described as 'oil-free and non-comedogenic'. Some products described as 'oil-free' actually contain silicone-based ingredients designed to prevent the colour pigment 'drifting' – that is, changing colour on the skin – but the more expensive oil-free products are more likely to be stable. These foundations are usually in liquid or lotion form.

Also, be aware that topical spot creams and medicated concealers may also cause the colour of your foundation to change.

Other foundations are described as 'oil-controlled'; this refers to the level of 'fillers' added to the product. These fillers play an important role in cosmetics suitable for those with oily or combination skins. They absorb excess oil produced by the skin, allowing the makeup to stay put longer. The most common oil-controlled foundations are water-based, liquid foundations.

CHOOSING YOUR FOUNDATION MAKEUP

Ask advice from the assistants on the cosmetics counter, but always test the foundation – on your neck instead of on the wrist or the back of the hand, as we're generally accustomed to doing! Use the mirror usually provided on the counter, or take one with you, and don't be afraid to walk out into the daylight to get a sense of the colour away from artificial light.

Since this is the most important, and perhaps most expensive item in your makeup collection, it's worth trying before you buy. So when you think you've decided on a product, apply a little of the colour you think best suits your skin to a test area, and wear it for the rest of the day to see how it behaves on your skin.

It's generally worth paying more for your base foundation than for other elements of your makeup. Splash out on the foundation and look for good but cheaper brands of eye make-up, for instance.

HOW TO APPLY FOUNDATION

Professional makeup artists use little sponges to apply foundation, rather than fingers. These wedge-shaped fine-pored sponges are available in packs from good makeup stores and they do produce a professional finish – but clean fingers can do as good a job.

Some cosmetics manufacturers offer makeup lessons, or makeovers at their counters in department stores, and it's interesting to watch one of these, even if you aren't brave enough to sit in a busy shop having your own face made up!

Many women's magazines have a regular reader's makeover feature. Useful tips for your own makeup, as well as up-to-date fashion styles, can always be picked up from these features.

Setting Powders and Blushers

Whatever foundation you use, the staying power of the base will only be as good as the setting of the foundation. Setting powder comes in 'cake' (compressed) form, or as loose powder. Makeup artists always use the loose form, but a compact of compressed powder is useful for touching-up during the day or before an evening out.

For anyone with an oily complexion, it's important to learn how to set your foundation in order for it to last as long as possible. Powdering gives the makeup a matte finish. Apply with a velour pad and whisk off the excess with a powder brush. Again these velour pads, or puffs, must be kept scrupulously clean.

A common mistake is to use powder as a blotter for a shiny face. This only results in a darkening of the makeup over the oily area, in particular, and could cause pore blockage and blackheads.

Blushers for the face are generally, nowadays, in powder form, which is applied after foundation and powder. They can be used to 'shape' the face or add a youthful, healthy glow. But don't be tempted to use too much! And always blend and shade it – rather than dabbing a circle of colour on your cheeks so that you resemble a china doll!

For applying blusher effectively, a professional domed blusher brush is a great deal more effective than the tiny squared brush often supplied by the manufacturer.

Indeed, investing in a good, basic set of makeup brushes is worthwhile for anyone who wants to make the most of their makeup.

Some acne sufferers find the use of a blusher brush leads to a breakout on the cheeks. If this happens use cream blush (rouge), a tinted colour wash, or bronzer, instead.

Eye Makeup

Eye makeup has been worn since the time of the Pharaohs. Drawing attention to the eyes can be a way of distracting attention from less than perfect skin in other areas of the face.

Colours of eyeshadow change with fashion, but no matter the colours featured in the fashion magazines, the standard charcoals, greys, browns and taupes still provide the most flattering effects. Colours providing contrast to the eye colour, such as the deeper plums, can be used to great effect, as can blue and green shadows – but subtlety is more effective than over-emphasis!

Muted shades can also enhance eye colours. Warm browns enrich blue eyes, gunmetal greys contrast brown eyes, whilst darker charcoal colours flatter green eyes.

Makeup artists always use sable brushes for eye makeup and, once you learn to use a proper brush instead of the stubby little, sponge-ended sticks often provided with eye shadow, you'll realize why!

Mascara and pencil eyeliners are often a problem for those with oily skin; waterproof mascaras and quick-drying eyeliner pens are the answer. Mascara sold for people who use contact lenses is also worth trying.

Lips and Lipsticks

For those with oily skin it's advisable to carry the foundation over the lip line and set with face powder. Lip bases or sealers are worth trying, and lip pencils are good for defining the lip line and can be used to provide a secure base for lipstick.

Makeup artists' advice for keeping lip and eye pencils sharp: Leave them in the fridge before sharpening!

And learn to use a lip brush! With practice the technique improves lipstick's lasting power. Lipstick can be set by blotting the lips carefully with a tissue.

Makeup Removers and Cleansers

It's important to remove your makeup at the end of each day, not only to remove dirt and grime from the atmosphere, but to remove loose skin cells. And it's more effective to remove makeup with a cleansing cream or lotion before washing the face. Choose an oil-free lotion or gel makeup remover which is designed for 'sensitive' or 'oily' skins and is non-comedogenic.

Facial Skin Care for Men

Cleansing

The basic advice, as above, applies both to men and women. Look for the words 'gentle', 'for sensitive skin', 'non-allergenic', or more upfront, 'non-comedogenic' on packaging of cleansing or washing soaps, gels and lotions.

Shaving

Shaving is often uncomfortable for men with acne and care should be taken to avoid undue damage to the pustules.

Most skin damage occurs when correct shaving methods are not followed. Shaving foams and gels are designed to provide lubrication between the razor blades and the skin. They also act to hydrate the hair shaft, causing it to swell and soften. This makes the hair far easier to cut, giving a smoother and less traumatic shave. This softening of the hair shaft takes around five minutes after application of the foam or gel.

Some of the aerosol foams on the market will begin to break down quite quickly on the skin. Shaving gels have better stability and many contain products such as aloe vera to soothe the skin.

The razor itself should be wetted in cold water prior to shaving and rinsed at regular intervals throughout the shave to remove the shaving products and cut hairs from the razor edge. The cutting edge of the razor should be kept clean at all times during the shave, as this greatly reduces the drag across the skin that is otherwise needed to cut the hairs. This drag gives rise to razor burn.

The newer flexible bladed razors have foils so supple that they bend and mould to the contours of your skin. This makes the blades far less likely to cut the skin than a fixed foil razor, and provide an even closer shave.

WET SHAVING

Use a moisturizer before shaving if your skin is dry. Wet the face before applying the shaving gel and make sure you leave the gel on the skin for at least five minutes before shaving. Shave with the direction of the hair growth. Don't stretch the skin too much. Use a sharp razor blade otherwise you will have to use too much force to cut the hairs and will certainly cause razor burn or other damage to the skin.

If you use an aftershave lotion, choose one designed for sensitive skin, with a low alcohol content.

ELECTRIC SHAVING

Electric shavers are, by comparison, far easier to use than a wet razor. A pre-electric shave lotion designed for sensitive skins is often helpful. These have the opposite effect to shaving foams and gels, by stripping the outer hair shaft of sebum and reducing internal moisture, making it more brittle and thus easily trimmed by the vibrating or spinning cutting blades of the electric shaver.

These pre-shave lotions do contain alcohol to dry out the hairs but may also contain silicone to prevent the skin from damage by its drying effect during shaving.

The cutters are prevented from touching and cutting the skin by a thin foil, and therefore cuts to the skin are reduced.

However, just as with a wet razor, the electric razor should be cleaned out regularly to prevent the internal mechanisms becoming clogged with cut hairs, thereby reducing the efficiency of the cutting action and causing greater shaving pressure to be applied in order to achieve a close shave. This increased pressure can lead to razor burn and follicular irritation, which in turn can lead to acne.

Moisturizers

Moisturizers are as important for men as for women, and come in many specially-designed products.

For Men and Women

Bronzers

Bronzing creams or gels give the skin the appearance of a natural tan, with the healthy look of an outdoor life without the risks associated with over-exposure to UV light. A tan enhances both male and female bodies, and many of the creams and lotions provide all the lubricant qualities of a standard moisturizer.

These products contain a transparent colour agent that stains the outer surface of the skin. This stain will, of course, also transfer onto your fingers when massaging the tinted moisturizer into the skin. It should be washed off your hands as soon as possible after application of the gel. Leave the bronzing gel for at least 10 minutes before bringing the skin into contact with clothing or bed linen.

Do make sure you choose a bronzing gel that enhances your natural skin colour. If your skin is a warm colour, choose a warm brown tint, if you turn a more golden tan in summer, choose a golden brown bronzer.

These bronze tints are simply washed off the skin at the end of each day.

Self-tanning Products

A semi-permanent tan (lasting for between three and four days) may be obtained with self-tanning lotions and creams. These products can be used on all parts of the body. They are very effective on those with sallow or golden skin tones, but less so for those with olive or dark skins.

The product is applied in a similar fashion to a moisturizer, taking care to avoid the eyebrows and also the hairline. The active ingredient in the self-tanning cream reacts with amino acids and other amino groups present in the keratin of the skin, resulting in a 'tan' that develops over several hours. As keratin is also found in the hair, similar staining may occur. This is particularly noticeable in fair-haired people.

Areas of the body which have a slightly more horny keratin layer, such as the elbows, knees, heels and knuckles, may also turn a darker colour than the rest of the skin. This is why a thinner layer of cream should be applied to these areas.

Those with blackheads or otherwise invisible blocked pores may also find that the active ingredient in self-tanning creams colours the small keratinized plug at the top of the follicle. This can result in an unattractive pitted appearance.

When using either bronzing gels or self-tanning products, make sure you apply the cream evenly – remembering to cover all exposed areas of skin to create a realistic tan. And don't forget the ears and the back of the neck!

It is important to stress that bronzing and self-tanning products provide no increased protection against natural or artificial UV rays. Many products contain sun-screen additives. However, it is vital to ensure that the level of protection (SPF) is adequate for the strength of the sun, the time of day – and your skin.

10

Facing Up to It

From Anger and Despair . . .

These are quotes from letters and telephone calls from acne sufferers:

I feel desperate and very depressed. All I know is what I see in the mirror – but I don't want to look any more. It embarrasses me and I've become very withdrawn. I have no social life.

I've lost my social life to acne. I've never had a girlfriend – girls stare at me. I often feel like suicide. I work at a burger bar but the managers don't want me on the tills. They say it 'scares customers away'.

It's exploded since my twenties. I've tried everything. Sometimes I cry with frustration. I feel humiliated.

Acne controls my life 100 per cent. I can't help picking the spots, which makes them worse so I have to have time off work. But I feel if I pick my face, maybe I'll get the badness out.

I feel I'm being punished for something.

After two hospitalizations for depression and self-injury, my life hasn't been taken over [by acne], but the spots do make things difficult.

From the age of 11, I avoided swimming at school and medicals. At 12, I was beaten up and called 'an abortion'. At 13 I covered my back with neat disinfectant and burned the skin. But all these experiences [this person is now 28] can make you a stronger person. I believe I am strong now.

My sister was beautiful – and I had acne. I had good academic results but I was too shy to go to university. I work in a shop. It took me four months to find the courage to go to a doctor. I watch the look on people's faces as they come near me.

I feel I'm cursed.

I hardly ever go out. I no longer work. I spend my day cleansing, washing, taking vitamins, drinking water and putting on creams and lotions. I squeeze obsessively. It's hopeless.

My boyfriend says he likes me the way I am. He says everyone has spots, but I don't think they do. I never let him see me without makeup.

All hell erupts on my face if I stop the medication.

I know nothing's going to work.

I don't go out in daylight. I avoid people. I feel disgusted with myself. What am I living for?

There's a lot of anger – and pain. It makes me feel ill. The pain wakes me up at night and keeps me awake with the throbbing. And when the spots are very deep it's difficult to eat.

Spots – who needs 'em!

Many people feel that acne has changed their lives. Some feel it has ruined it. At the very least, they feel they have become different people because of it, or they have missed chances or let opportunities slip away because of the way they've felt about themselves and the way they look.

Most admit that they probably notice the spots more than other people do, but when other people say, 'They're not too bad' or 'It really doesn't show all that much' they feel doubtful and suspect they're just being pacified, or even patronized.

Most people who suffer from acne are more self-conscious about themselves and the spots than others around them – family, lovers and friends – will allow. This often compounds the problem.

A typical acne sufferer's comment is, 'I'd say I was quite obsessed by acne. It's the first thing I think of every morning when I wake up, and looking to see what my face is like is the first thing I do. It's just habit – and if it isn't too bad – I feel glad. It's just what I do.'

Consultant psychologist Aric Sigman, talking to *Face Forward*, the magazine of the Acne Support Group, says –

Acne strikes when people are growing up, in the formative, teenage years. You're forming a self-image and your face is the expression of that image. When you study it in the mirror, you're assessing your sexual attractiveness in the market place. To be affected in the formative years means that the damage isn't going to go away. It sickens me to think that acne is trivialized. To have huge scars on your face for five to ten years and to be told that growing up is a difficult time isn't far from impossible to cope with.

The people who cope with it best, Dr Sigman says, are the ones who 'have an information base and are taking action'. 'It's the act of doing something that's terribly important'.

A young woman in her late twenties agrees:

A turning point for me was educating myself. Once I understood that it was a hormonal thing and it wasn't anything to do with me, that was good for me. I also started talking to people and telling them why I felt ill and miserable.

Anger about Acne

As Aric Sigman says, 'Anger isn't a "bad" emotion. But feeling angry isn't a pleasant feeling. Expressing anger is a good way of diminishing it.'

The anger around acne is caused by the difference between what you want – that is, a reasonably clear complexion – and what you actually have.

All your attempts at doing something about the problem are frustrated. Nothing works. It feels like a conspiracy against you and you feel that you alone have been singled out to be in this position.

All this comes at a time when you feel you have to be as attractive as possible because you've got to start dealing with the opposite sex. And it's one extra burden – an enormous burden – which at this time you just don't need. Adolescence is bad enough without this too!

You're influenced by all the advertisements on TV and in magazines, which promise you a clear skin. You pay out a lot of money – (the most recent marketing figures estimated a sum of £94,000 being spent each day in Britain on skin-clearing products) – and often they don't work!

You feel helpless. You find yourself in what psychologists call a 'state of learned helplessness' and the deeper you've dived into it, the more difficult it is to extricate yourself.

An Action Plan

It's essential to start taking some action. You need to have a plan of action – to try to find some sense of control over your own skin and over your own life.

Once you feel you've regained some control, the anger should lessen.

One essential element of this action plan is to feel you're getting proper treatment and some significant help for your acne.

Talk

You need to talk to people who have a complete understanding of acne, and to get away from those who are making 'false promises' and whose interest in your skin is merely to take money from you.

You need to find sympathetic and empathetic help, and talking to others who share your experiences is a positive help. People like the Acne Support Group can make all the difference – on the basis that 'a problem shared is a problem halved.'

Talking to family, partners and close friends about the way you feel can be positive as long as they react positively.

But beware of talking inappropriately, in the sense of acne becoming a personal, political statement of yourself, instead of a skin condition.

There is a 'school of victimology' which separates people out into categories because they are, for example, from a different racial group, they're without a limb, they're working class, homosexual ... or whatever. This isn't helpful. It's saying, 'I am deficient in some way and I want to let you know about it. I want to use it as a form of identity.'

By crusading on a 'victimhood' platform, you're elevating a skin condition to a level it may well not justify. You're redefining yourself as some sort of victim. You've become 'a person with acne', instead of 'a person'.

When Life Doesn't Seem Worth Living

A fair number of letters to the Acne Support Group talk of a level of desperation which is frightening. For some people, the struggle to cope with acne has become more than they can bear. It seems to be affecting every part of their life and taking over.

When life feels hopeless, remember the Samaritans. (There is one national number to call – 0345 90 90 90.)

Samaritans are used to talking with people about every problem known to humanity.

'Ian', a London Samaritan, remembers a conversation with a young woman whose feelings about her acne were threatening to overwhelm her – and not for the first time.

She talked – and he listened – and their conversation is typical of the sort of help Samaritans offer to anyone who feels they're reaching a point where they're unable to cope with life and its problems.

She's apologetic about calling – but feels there's nowhere else to turn. She's embarrassed about feeling so bad about something which isn't life-threatening, but which sometimes makes her feel like ending it all.

She feels ugly – as if she's touched by the plague. If she says this to family or friends, they try to brush it off, saying things like, 'They're not too bad – and you've got such pretty hair and a good figure ...'

This only makes her feel more alone with her problem – that nobody understands or is prepared to listen to what she says about the depths of her distress.

She feels disregarded – that people aren't taking her, or her acne, seriously.

This not only applies to family and friends – but also to her doctor. She feels he thinks she's pestering him, and when she goes back for more prescriptions she feels he's irritated with her – which sometimes makes her reluctant to ask why the treatment doesn't seem to be working – and sometimes just makes her angry and hurt. None of which helps her skin condition!

When it is at its worst she says she feels out of control of her life, as if her acne is eating up her life – as well as, somehow, eating up her face. In her case, the acne also affects the skin on her back and chest and, consequently, she feels unable to wear clothes which expose these parts of her body, in summer or in the evening. She feels she has to hide under her clothes – which in itself exacerbates the feeling that the acne is controlling her life and imprisoning her against her will.

Sometimes this makes her feel very low, or depressed – which of course means different things to different people. It can make you feel withdrawn and increase the feeling of isolation from the rest of the world – which seems, when you're in this sort of state, to be universally happy and spot-free!

As a Samaritan, Ian had to ask if she had ever felt suicidal. But for this young woman, her depression was more a feeling of a burden which was constantly with her, on her shoulder or weighing her down – but which she had to carry while she continued with everyday life, going to work and – in her case – looking after her young daughter.

Ian remarked to her that different people have different reactions to depression – and in some cases, it can make you feel very angry. He asked if she felt angry – and she agreed – vehemently!

Anger can be useful in some ways, Ian told her, in that it gives vent to some of the feelings of frustration that are also common for people suffering from a disfiguring skin condition.

The frustration arises from the feeling that you're powerless against the condition – that it's winning and taking over your life – and the feelings of powerlessness in themselves make you feel angry and bitter.

Of course, he said, this can affect your relationships with the people around you – especially if you feel they're not doing their best to understand you and your distress, or are not giving you the help you need and deserve – as can sometimes be the case with doctors.

But it can also affect relationships in ways that are unreasonable.

This woman said she felt she was irritable and short-tempered at work – which she knew was unfair on her colleagues and could even jeopardize her employment.

But, even worse, she felt she sometimes took her anger about her acne out on her young daughter – which she hated in herself.

Ian asked if that was the root of the matter, in a sense. That she hated herself.

When her acne was really bad, she agreed that she did hate herself or, at least, she hated the way she looked.

But, as Ian said – the way we look on the outside isn't what we are. Realizing this and coming to terms with it is a step on the road to coming to terms with the problem of acne.

This young woman said she'd needed to talk to someone who'd listen – and not judge her – and to think about what was troubling her.

Talking like this can be a way of putting a new perspective on your feelings and your life at the moment.

Just by saying things to someone which you've only thought, but never said, before, helps to take some of the agony out of the feeling. It's as if, by saying them – putting them into the air – they become somehow less destructive and less fearsome.

It may never have occurred to you that you feel bad enough to telephone the Samaritans. But they are not just for people who feel suicidal. They are for people at crisis point – and it doesn't matter how big or how relatively small the crisis is. If it feels like a crisis for you – it's serious.

You might find that a conversation like this could be enough to give you courage and renewed strength to keep you going.

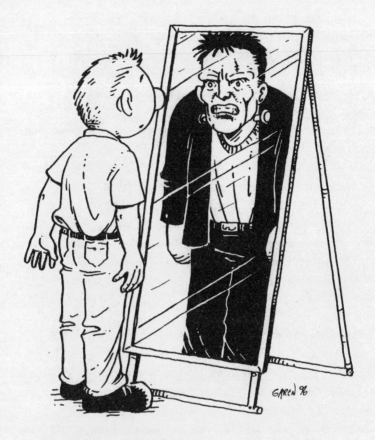

The Way You See Yourself

If you hate the way you look to yourself in the mirror, you imagine that others see you – in the street or wherever you go out and about – in the same way. The fact they probably don't is of no interest!

If you hate the way you look, you're likely to hate the way you feel about yourself and find it hard to make connections with other people, or to develop relationships with them.

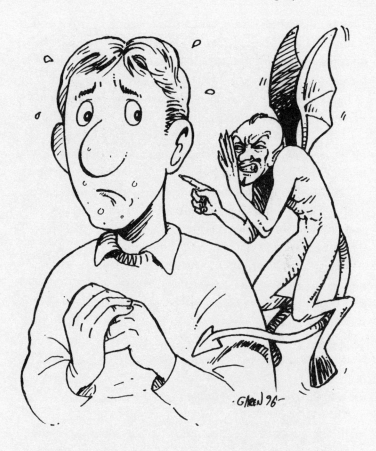

'DEMONS'

It's as if there's a 'demon' on your shoulder, whispering in your ear – 'Why should anyone want to look at me, or talk to me, or make friends with me? I'm ugly and horrible.'

We have to contend with all sorts of 'demons' like this, in life. Demons tell us things that undermine and threaten us. They travel with us all through life, from our earliest days.

They begin with a word or an idea or a feeling in childhood. If someone tells you when you're six years old that you can't do sums – you can't add up – you might well believe you're hopeless with numbers all your life.

If, at around the same time, someone either at home or school says you aren't very clever or even that you are 'stupid' – you might also believe this too and it might stay with you for a very long time, buried under the layers of confidence you might cover yourself with as you grow up and grow older.

The 'little demon' sits there quite quietly, sometimes for years at a time, until something happens to you or someone says something to you – when it leaps up onto your shoulder and says, 'There, I always told you you were – (stupid/ugly/useless, etc.)!'

Often this happens when you least expect it. You've been going along quite happily through life, behaving like a competent, mature adult. Then all of a sudden you do something, or say something – and you're a small child again, feeling as you did then – feeling stupid. It's a horrible feeling.

If you have been told – or have somehow been given the impression – that you're not a pretty or attractive child, this too will be likely to stay with you all your life.

If you're obviously 'different' – with a deformity, malformation or disfigurement that's plain to see, especially on your face – you will have to work harder than anyone else to handle the way you feel about yourself and the way you think others feel about you.

People with acne can identify with people who suffer disfigurement for other reasons – because acne can certainly leave disfiguring scars on the face and on the body which affect and 'disfigure' the mind in a similar way.

Changing Faces

Changing Faces is a charity dedicated to offering 'a better future for facially disfigured people'. It was set up in 1992 by James Partridge, whose face was badly burned in a car accident when he was 18. As part of its service, it offers workshops for groups of people who are facially disfigured in some way. The workshops aim to help them come to terms with themselves and learn skills to cope with the difficulties of life in a world where your 'looks' are considered all-important. 'Looks' can make the difference between getting a job and being turned down for it – or between getting a girlfriend – or boyfriend – or being rejected.

It's hard to unlearn the thinking that tells you that the way you look is the way you are – but that's what has to be done if you are to make life work for you instead of letting life get you down.

Learning to Re-think

The workshops run by Changing Faces are intended to help people gain confidence in themselves and in their ability to manage other people's reaction to them.

The basic principles of positive communication skills – encompassing confidence-building and assertiveness – are useful tools for everyone to acquire as they affect every part of life. But for those who feel disadvantaged – and are, in fact, disadvantaged by something about them that causes them to be visually different from the 'commonplace', these skills can mean the difference between a positive, fulfilling life and unhappiness or depression.

There is an old Spanish proverb, which was quoted in the Australian film *Strictly Ballroom*: 'A life lived in fear is a life half-lived.'

If we live in constant fear, with the expectation of being rejected – or stared at – we live with our eyes down, our shoulders hunched, and we stand little or no chance of looking life in the face and making the most of it.

Learning confidence-building skills and being encouraged to use them in everyday life can make all the difference.

This is true for anyone, whether or not they have a problem with acne.

Building Confidence

The following is taken – with very grateful thanks – from the worksheets provided for Changing Faces workshop participants.

Effective interpersonal communication comes from using all our verbal and non-verbal equipment in a consistent way. Speaking without expression is unlikely to convince anyone that you are an imaginative person – and similarly, walking with eyes down and rounded, shoulders dropped, sends negative, defensive messages.

The REACH OUT model involves bringing verbal and non-verbal language into positive action. The general principles can then be used together or in various combinations, to tackle specific 'difficult' situations.

REACH OUT stands for:

R – Reassuring – the other person, with a first impression of a smile, eye contact or a handshake. It means taking the initiative in the interchange instead of watching and waiting for the other's reaction.

E – Engaging – those we meet without the assumption of rejection. The temptation to back away at the first sign of uncertainty or rejection can be overcome by extra EFFORT.

A – Asserting – our right to be treated with respect. The use of communication equipment such as tone of voice and eye contact can help to convince a potential threat of the strength of our position.

C – Courage – to take up the challenge. You can show this by standing firm and upright – holding your head high.

H – Humour – to laugh at ourselves and to see the funny side of ourselves. The use of words, pitch and tone can make humour from the tiniest morsel. Humour is a powerful weapon and can also be used as armour.

O – 'Otherness' – replacing self-consciousness with consciousness of the other person, shifting attention from yourself to someone or something else.

U – Understanding – An awareness of how the other person might be feeling.

T – Tenacity, or Try again ... Don't give up without giving it another go.

THE REACH OUT STRATEGY, STEP BY STEP

1 It's disarming – and positively advantageous – to take the initiative in an interchange or a meeting. It puts you in charge – on top. Smile immediately and make eye contact with the other person. Say something – 'hello' is a good place to start! Introduce yourself – 'I'm ... – it takes the emphasis off you and puts it onto them. Offer your hand, if appropriate, in greeting.

2 Make a positive connection – or engagement – with another person with the assumption and presumption that they will

make a similar engagement with you. Avoiding the assumption that they will ignore, overlook or reject you. Believe, at the same time, that if they do any of these – it's their problem – and you needn't bother too much about them. You wouldn't want to know them anyway!

3 Assert your basic human right to respect from another human being. Use a confident tone of voice and friendly, open manner – likewise body language. Use a bit of effort and energy to do this – which adds conviction to the whole effect.

4 Courage and conviction. It takes guts to start on this course of assertive confidence – especially if you've slipped into 'bad habits' of feeling and looking shy and embarrassed in social situations – but the more you do it, the more courage you will acquire. And you can practise in private at first – in front of a mirror. You'll feel stupid at first – but who cares?! Then you can practise in 'easier' situations, such as:
   – saying 'good morning' to the bus driver as you get on
   – making a remark about the weather (well why not?) to the person next to you as you wait in the bus queue. It doesn't matter if they don't reply!
   – asking for directions to somewhere nearby
   – asking for directions for somewhere more complicated.
   If you practise regularly – daily at least – it will gradually feel safer and less threatening to make contact with people in everyday life.

5 Humour is a great face-saver. It can also be used as a defence. How often have you read biographies of famous comedians and heard how they developed a sense of humour – became a 'fool' – to defend themselves against ridicule or persecution because they were smaller than average (for some reason this seems to be very common for

comedians) – or always bottom of the class, or no good at games, or looked funny?

If witty one-liners don't come naturally to you, either rehearse one or two humorous responses to common remarks – or learn how to turn round a situation to laugh at yourself. But beware! There is a danger that humour can become irony – which can become sarcasm, used as a defensive barrier against communication. If you use humour to put others down – because you find you can – you will inevitably make more enemies than friends!

One man, who'd become bald through alopecia – but who always chose to pretend his hairdo was the latest style statement – was a natural wit. But he'd begun to realize he'd gone a bit too far the other side of humour, towards sarcasm and bitterness, when he saw that this defence mechanism had become a barrier between him and the world – and especially women, who perhaps find it less easy to understand this type of wisecrack.

So use humour with good-natured care! Look for the funny side of life.

6 Turning self-consciousness into 'other-consciousness'. This is a rather clumsy way of making the point that if you're so taken up with thinking about yourself, how you look and appear to others, and imagining what they're thinking of you – you can't possibly be taking notice of them! You can't listen properly to what someone is saying to you – so you can't make or take part in a conversation. You may also appear inattentive, or stupid – which is the last thing you intend!

Lots of books have been written about how to cope with shyness, because millions of people in this world suffer from the problem! It isn't only you! Not everyone, by any means, finds it easy, for instance, to walk into a room full of people on their own, or make conversation with someone they've just met – let alone face a job interview or speak in public.

There are skills you can learn to help manage all these situations – but the first step is to get out of the habit of concentrating on yourself and concentrate on the other person, or people.

You have to shift the focus – and a good, well-tried way of doing that is to use what are called 'open questions'. These are conversational questions which invite an informative reply – instead of merely a yes or a no. Picking up on something someone's wearing – clothing, jewellery – is an easy way. It isn't rude to give a compliment – 'I like your earrings, necklace, coat, hat ... where did it/they come from? (And incidentally – let's get out of the habit of putting down this sort of compliment with a 'What, this old thing? How much more friendly and civilized to say, 'Thank you – yes I like it/them too, a friend gave them to me/found them in a junk shop – it came from ...')

By conversing in this way, you established a frame of reference – a similar or like opinion or taste which makes it easier to go on with the conversation. If you've made the effort and the approach and shifted the emphasis in the way we've been discussing – and you get a negative response: don't give up – give it one more try. If you still can't make headway, then maybe write that one off as a no-no.

Which brings us to:

7 Alongside the knack of flipping the coin and putting the other person in the spotlight – becoming other-conscious instead of self-conscious – is the skill of putting yourself into the other person's shoes. Try to understand and

imagine how they're feeling. Empathy is the word for this. If they're feeling uneasy, nervous and embarrassed too, you can understand this and even use this as a way of communicating and sharing – and helping you both to relax.

8 Tenacity – not giving up. As the old saying goes, 'If at first you don't succeed, try, try again.' Another cliché is 'Practice makes perfect.' To put it in more modern terms, 'There is no such thing as failure – only feedback.'

This may call for a little explanation. It's about never allowing yourself to describe an incident as a 'failure' but talking yourself through it, looking at what happened and working out what could have been done, or said, better. So when you miss an opportunity of picking up on an opening someone has made for you – and perhaps only realize afterwards and wish you'd said something different – don't leave it on a downbeat. Work out what you might have said, or done, and store it away in your mind for another time.

The first time you recognize that you've made a change in yourself and your behaviour, it'll give you a little more courage to try again and make another change, or take another step.

Confidence can be learned. To begin with it can be an act, or a performance, and for many of us it always is. But it's possible for it to give such a convincing performance that you believe in it yourself.

You may find that this confidence can be dented, even after many years of practice, when something unexpected happens. Perhaps someone says something unkind and unnecessary, or you're just having a bad day and everything goes wrong. But it doesn't matter. You can always go back and recover the situation in your 'feedback', for next time.

Courses and Training

Becoming more confidently assertive is about learning the difference between assertion and aggression, activity and passivity, and positive and negative behaviour. It's sometimes as simple as using different words and language in ordinary (but sometimes difficult) everyday situations, either in our 'public' life or in our 'private' personal relationships.

It's about dealing with situations as diverse as returning faulty goods to the shop where they were bought, asking the neighbours to turn down their music, or telling a friend, or lover, you'd rather stay in tonight and watch TV than go out with them.

Assertion Training

Many adult education institutes now include assertiveness training in their prospectus, sometimes in separate gender groups and sometimes in mixed ones. And there are also many self-help books on the subject.

Some people learn easily from a book, while others find it better to learn as part of a group. One advantage of a group is that you can learn from each other's experiences – as well as finding a possible source of new friendships.

To start you thinking about assertiveness, read a booklet published by MIND, called 'How to Assert Yourself'. This explains the basic principles, with examples of how to use them in everyday social and relationship situations.

You Can Change

In this chapter we've progressed, as it were, from darkness into light.

It is certainly possible for anyone, with some energy and determination, to change the way they think about themselves and the way they behave, in relation to themselves and to others.

11

You and Your Relationships

You are you.

You're not your acne!

At bad times you may begin to feel there's nothing more important in your life than the way your skin looks. But that's a dangerous – and negative – attitude to adopt, and one that won't make you happy or improve your relationships.

Parents and Close Family

Most parents worry about their children all the time, but worry about them most when they can see they are unhappy.

Many mothers have written to the Acne Support Group begging for help for their son or daughter, because they don't know where to turn.

One mother wrote in about her 23-year old son:

He's handsome, intelligent with a good degree, but I feel that some of his best years have been ruined by acne. His self-esteem is low, he has no confidence, meeting new people is agony for him.

This woman goes on to say, however, that her son now has a girlfriend 'who seems to love him whatever his skin does'. So perhaps this young man's girlfriend doesn't notice the spots as much as his mother does!

Parents can be positively supportive, by helping with the perseverance often necessary in order to find the right treatment and by bolstering confidence, throughout their child's life, with solid, background reassurance that he or she is loved and respected. But they can sometimes be less of a help and more of a real hindrance. As one Acne Support Group member recalls:

My dad used to come out with comments such as 'stop picking your pimples.' I hated my acne being called 'pimples'. It was almost as if I had an enemy in the home as well as the enemy of acne. Because it was his ignorance of acne and his ignorance of my feelings which was belittling. If he saw me eating chocolate I'd be given 'that look'. You know ... 'you shouldn't be eating and enjoying that' ... which I think it's fair to say is a common reaction from family and friends.

And another young woman in her late twenties says:

My mother encouraged me to go back to the doctor when I was 18, and thought it would never go away. Ten years later, though she's very supportive and kind, I don't think she really understands that it's an illness. My sister and brother had acne – but they don't have it now. They 'grew out of it' as my parents expected, but I still have it.

How They Can Help

Talk to your parents and tell them what action you're taking to get help for your condition. Explain what you've discovered about acne, and pass on the information to them so they understand – at whatever level they're prepared to reach. The more people who know the truth about acne, the better. This is the way that knowledge is spread.

If you're under 16, ask a parent to come with you to the doctor if you think that will give you support and encourage the doctor to take more notice of you. But you don't have to go to a doctor with a parent or guardian. You're entitled to confidential information and treatment with or without a parent's knowledge.

Friends

What do you say to people? There's nothing more frustrating than when other people tell me about their spots. But I'm obsessed with looking at other people's skin. I get very envious.

My face erupted. And there was a huge spot right by my eye and it was all I could see. I was working at an employment agency at the time and the girls there were lovely – I could talk to them about it. But once one of them was moaning about a spot on her chin and I said – Sonia, don't you know what I'd give just to have one spot! And I really laid into her. I think at last they realized how sensitive I was about it. But that day I asked to move to the back of the room because I felt so self-conscious about my face. The manageress asked me why and I burst into tears and everyone got very emotional. That was the worst time.

Two descriptions from two young women with different, but comparably unfortunate experiences of reactions from friends and work colleagues. In fact, it seems there is an almost universal hatred – not too strong a word – of comments which 'put down' or apparently dismiss a sufferer's acne as 'not too bad'.

If you've learned something about self-confidence and assertiveness, you can cope better with this sort of well-meaning but insensitive comment. But it's worth telling friends with whom you're close enough to be straightforward – or whose friendship you value – why you feel upset by what they've said, and then ask to talk about it. Again, that's how the rest of the world learns how to deal with acne.

The Difference Between Boys and Girls

Psychologist Aric Sigman takes the view that there is a different perception of 'spots' between boys and girls, or men and women.

Girls have a different perception of what the acne looks like to boys. The spots for girls are physically smaller.

Acne spots are worse for a boy than for a girl. There's 15 times more testosterone, for a start, which makes it worse. And boys can't cover them up with makeup either.

For a girl, any kind of deviation from a completely smooth skin is awful – but it's awful in relative terms. The way it looks to boyfriends – to men – or perhaps to people in general – is really quite negligible. There's an enormous difference between what girls think boys notice – and what they actually notice. So a girl might think a boy is looking at the spot on her face – when actually he's looking down her shirt, or imagining what's underneath. There's a discrepancy there and one that's worth being aware of.

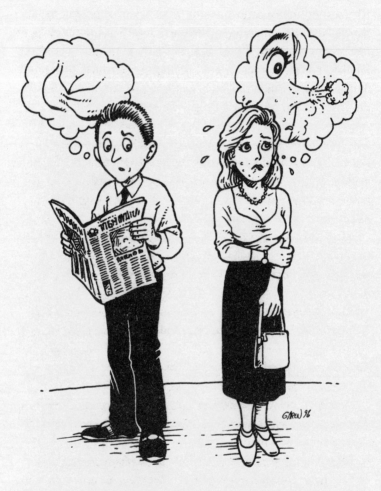

In general, anyway, boys are much less observant than girls. It's the same with the way girls notice changes in their own weight. Boys and men don't notice these subtle changes and they don't care. They wouldn't notice the odd half-stone [5–7 lb], for instance – in fact they'd probably prefer a bit more weight on a girl. They'd notice extremes – of course – but not small changes.

Nick Fisher, advice columnist for *Just 17* magazine agrees that boys suffer worse than girls with their acne because 'They have fewer ways of coping – less means of taking the pressure off, of talking about it or even of getting filial support from their mates.' And, in his experience, teenage girls and boys remark on acne in each other in different ways.

A girl will say of another girl – 'she's got bad spots.' Whereas a boy would never say something like that about a girl. It would be much lower down the list of things he would judge her by. He'd be far more likely to make comments about her size – for instance – than about her skin.

Boys ... out of sheer boredom, will search for a scapegoat – someone to pick on – and a boy with acne will be the one. Of course, boys are much more competitively aggressive with each other than girls are.

Boys will often attack spots in not particularly helpful ways. Their own – and others. They'll attack each other's spots – physically – a boy will try to squeeze another boy's spots on his neck – and of course verbally, by being abusive.

Boys aren't good at knowing what to do about a problem like acne. They don't know where to start – they don't know how to get a result. Girls are far better educated about anything medical or physical.

Girls have more chance of disguising their spots, too, and are better at it. If a boy puts a load of flesh-tinted cream on his spots he'll be risking setting himself up for a whole lot more abuse. He'll be taunted not only for having the spots but also for wearing 'makeup'!

A bit of acne is quite an attractive thing. It's a kind of acceptable flaw in a person. In the same way that slightly shy people can be very attractive – because the shyness puts the other person at their ease, by comparison, and they don't feel they have to try too hard with them.

Girls who are terribly attractive – stunningly beautiful – can be very off-putting to the average boy.

And of course, acne is always worse from the inside – than from the outside.

Hundreds of letters from acne sufferers tell of teasing and bullying at school because of the opportunity offered to the perpetrators by a spotty face or body. And the damage this sort of behaviour does to a person is much more than skin-deep.

We need supportive relationships around us – from the cradle to the grave – and when we're suffering, for any reason, or if we struggle with a long-term condition or illness, we need extra and perhaps more knowledgeable, skilful and sensitive support.

However, as much we love someone, sometimes it's difficult to know how to help and what they need – or don't need – from us.

Partners and Lovers

A letter from a man of 30, who has suffered with acne since the age of 13, begins 'I feel I'm cursed.' He goes on:

My wife has to put up with my weeks and sometimes months of moaning and the fact I will never move out of the house until my face is clear. She doesn't mind, but after several cancelled holidays and having to attend family functions alone, she's now at the end of her tether.

Another man, of 32, whose acne began only two years before, writes in desperation:

Yes, I'm stressed, but so is anyone with two young children and a mortgage! My wife has been understanding, however she now thinks I'm paranoid and I can't even discuss the problem with her. I'm so depressed. My personality has changed and I really don't go out any more.

The Effect on Relationships

Every relationship between two people is different – and complicated. And there is always a great deal else going on between them than, very often, they realize themselves.

Most of us have enough to do to cope with the everyday stresses of life, like working, looking after children, paying bills, making ends meet, as well as trying to manage and sustain a relationship. Anything else that adds to the stress can threaten to stretch it beyond breaking point – or sometimes can, in a strange way, prop up the relationship by giving the partners separate and supportive roles within it, without which neither feels needed.

There are some questions to be asked about the people involved in the previous two incidences, and how their relationships developed.

In the first case, the husband's acne seems to be dominating his life. He seems to want it to dominate and control his wife's life as well. He refuses to leave the house and his wife has been forced – or perhaps has been determined – to go out and do things without him. She can cope with 'family functions' alone – but holidays are more difficult. It's not surprising that after two cancellations she's getting fed up.

Obviously the acne is overwhelming him, but it is also giving him 'excuses' to refuse invitations and cancel plans – which might perhaps be a way of demanding attention from wife and family. This could be because of unmet needs in the marriage – which is one thing – but it could just as easily be as a result of the frustration felt by so many acne patients when medication doesn't work and treatments fail – or worse still, when doctors seem to be unable or unwilling to take the problem seriously.

In the second couple's case, it seems the husband's acne has changed his personality and led to severe depression. His wife, while at first wanting to be sympathetic, has run out of understanding and is struggling to remain in communication with him.

Living with someone who is depressed is a difficult and in itself deeply depressing experience. Depression is an illness which needs treatment and understanding – just as acne does. If the two are connected, a good, sensitive doctor will take notice of both and treat or refer each with equal concern. But it is worth being aware of the fact of depression, for the person who's suffering with acne as well as those living with and loving them.

If this is an issue for you or your partner or someone in the family, it's essential to talk about it. And talk to your doctor where appropriate. And ask for help.

HOW TO TELL IF YOU OR SOMEONE CLOSE TO YOU IS DEPRESSED:

Do they:

- seem constantly tired?
- go to bed but either don't sleep or wake up early in the morning?
- seem unable to take interest in anything?
- seem to have lost interest in things they previously enjoyed, including sex?

- want to stay in bed, or if they get up, don't bother to get dressed?
- fail to wash themselves, or their hair, or shave?
- seem increasingly irritable and short-tempered?

A combination of some or all of these signals is often an indication of a depressive condition which needs taking seriously.

Roles in Relationships

In personal, emotional and sexual relationships, we all play different roles. These can change throughout the development of the relationship and can be dependent on balancing our needs with those of our partner, or on demands made, consciously or unconsciously, in the relationship.

In the first couple's relationship quoted above, the husband is insisting on playing the major and dominant role in the marriage. He may have always played this role – or he may be using his acne to claim it from his wife.

In the second situation, the husband's acne and resultant change of personality has altered the whole basis of the relationship so that it could well threaten the family's future.

These are just two examples of the importance of seeing the person as a whole, within his or her world, and treating the condition with this in mind.

A Partner's Influence

A lady of 65 wrote to the Acne Support Group, to tell of her problems with acne throughout her adult life. She had been married for 41 years and was a grandmother several times over.

She said that her skin had improved after a hysterectomy which she had undergone as treatment for endometriosis, but she was still troubled by scarring. Her dermatologist had suggested dermabrasion but, she said, 'My husband is against it. He's always said, "leave well alone. It looks OK to me".' Consequently, she had not gone back to the dermatologist and done nothing about the scarring.

It might have been suggested that this woman reconsider her decision and perhaps break the pattern of a lifetime's marriage by disregarding her husband's opinion about how her face looks and taking more notice of how she herself feels about it!

Partners can sometimes be guilty of 'negative help' – in the interests of their own role in the relationship. Counsellors and psychotherapists often notice a pattern of support in a partnership where one person needs to be the support and prop of the other, in order to feel good about themselves. For instance, the wife whose husband left her soon after her speech impediment, a stutter, had been drastically improved by speech therapy. She had been so bad at times that she could not answer the telephone and her husband had got into the habit of negotiating all family and domestic matters for her. In effect, he'd become her voice. When the speech therapist helped his wife to manage her impediment so effectively that she began to be able to speak for herself, her husband found himself at a loss, felt useless, became impotent – and instead of making any attempt to understand the change and adapt their relationship accordingly, he took off. He needed her to be unable to communicate without him – and could not cope with her new-found skills and perhaps the confidence and happiness that went along with them.

Comparisons can be drawn with the couple who always came along together for the wife's appointments with the consultant dermatologist. She had been suffering badly with acne throughout the time they had been together, but was finally on the way to positive treatment. Her husband was encouraging and supportive throughout her six-month treatment, and helped her when she felt like giving up – so many patients experience this, during the times when it seems that the condition is getting worse before it eventually gets better.

At the end of the treatment, her skin was noticeably improved and she felt and looked better than she had done for years. But suddenly, her husband left her and they are now divorced.

Relationships are complicated and difficult at the best of times, and it's easy for a problem such as acne to become an important 'issue' between a couple.

Being a Partner

If you're in a relationship with someone who suffers from acne, and want to be helpful and supportive, you need to be aware of the problems and to sympathize even if you can never entirely know what it feels like.

A man who has been for three years the partner of a woman in her late twenties with acne has become very involved with her acne, as he has become involved in the rest of her life. He feels very strongly that not enough is known about the condition and how it affects sufferers, and is concerned to pass on his experience for the benefit of others.

When we met, the first thing I noticed about Jill was her eyes. She has lovely eyes. I can't quite remember whether Jill mentioned she had acne or whether it was when she suddenly had a bad bout that

I first noticed it. I think it was when she had trouble smiling because the acne was so painful. I asked her why she was smiling a bit oddly and she said, 'Because my face hurts'.

When someone tells me they're in pain, I take notice. I couldn't understand why acne could cause so much pain. I learned an incredible amount straightaway.

Before, like most people, I'd thought acne was due to a bad diet or greasy skin, that teenagers get it and then grow out of it. I didn't know there was a condition that caused acne and that Jill suffered from it in a different way from the way teenagers suffer.

I found it difficult at first because I couldn't do anything about the pain, and it all seemed so far away from what I knew. Now I know it's related to hormones, and Jill has to be on medication or it's much worse.

Up until then it hadn't affected 'us' – it hadn't affected Jill's moods. But sometimes when it's bad, you just can't cover it up. It affects her psychologically, emotionally and physically. So, as her partner, it affects us both – it affects 'our' mood.

At the beginning I was very aware Jill had acne – she was very aware of it – and what she needed was for me not to draw attention to it. But I was drawing attention to it because it's so visible. I was continually saying, 'Are you OK? – Is it any better?' That wasn't helping because it was reinforcing her self-consciousness. What she needed to hear was 'You look good – your eyes are lovely, your hair's nice – you look really pretty in that dress.' To divert attention from the problem.

I'm a practical person and I want to help. Jill's condition made me feel helpless and frustrated. And I must admit there was an element of wondering how it would affect us when we went out. Are people going to stare at Jill? Is she going to feel uncomfortable? Should we go out at all?

Sometimes, when it was bad, Jill didn't want to go out at all and that was frustrating for me because, at that time, she hadn't told many people what she was suffering from. I felt very differently. I felt she should tell people it wasn't the kind of acne they think they know about – but a real illness. Eventually she did – but it took a while and she found it very difficult.

Sometimes I'd tell people – our friends. Sometimes when we weren't together someone would say, 'Jill was quiet at the weekend,' and I'd say it was because she suffers from acne.

Usually our friends were interested, and sympathetic. We told our close friends, but then we stopped telling everyone because it wasn't an issue with people we didn't know so well.

But I still think talking about it is good, because it spreads the word and educates people.

There was a time, at the beginning, when Jill was very bad, when she said, 'Maybe we shouldn't see each other when I'm like this?' And tempting as it was because it's the easy option, I didn't want that to happen because I felt I'd be letting her down – and we'd deal with it together. Since we got through the first year or so, we've been OK!

But there are always going to be bad moments. I remember one of the worst was my first big party at work in my first year in this job. Jill had a bad bout and it did lead to arguments and frustrations for us both. But in the end we went to the party and Jill did a great makeup job and it was fine. She was still in pain – that doesn't go away – but we got through the party. Once you've done something like that it gets better for the next time. But it's a problem if, like for us, Jill's bad bouts are very sporadic. She'll go for six or seven months of nothing – I'll have worse spots than her! – and then it'll flare up – and you've forgotten how bad it can get. You have to learn all over again.

Jill isn't obsessed by her acne, but I think she is preoccupied by it. She's very aware of it and she'll go to any lengths, medically or whatever, within limits. But she has to live her life. She has to accept it as part of her life, until such time as there's a major change in her life

– like having a baby. I know there's no guarantee that would eliminate it – it could make it worse – but it could improve it.

She's very aware of the side-effects of the medication and anti-biotics and their possible effect on fertility. That's very important indeed for her – and it is for me, knowing how important childbearing will be for her when she's ready to do that.

I remember when Jill read an article about a woman in her fifties, still suffering from acne, who'd had similar experiences to hers, such as being in an important business meeting and knowing a spot was weeping or bleeding – feeling demeaned in front of her professional peers. It made her realize, I think for the first time, that she wasn't alone. That's how she heard about the Acne Support Group.

Knowing there's support from other people who know how she feels is an enormous help, because – as much support I can give her as her partner – I'll never know how she really feels, especially when she's going through a bad spell.

I often feel I could never do the things Jill does when her acne is bad! She goes out – goes to meetings, presentations and so on – and goes out with friends. And I know she's suffering – I know it looks bad – but she just gets on with it. I don't think I could do it. She seems to be saying, 'This is the way I am – you just have to like it or lump it!'

I feel protective of Jill – and defensive for her and for others who suffer from the effects of acne. I get very annoyed about things like TV advertisements for skin products and skin care showing beautiful women with perfect skin, saying, 'this is how I keep my skin clear.' They're rubbish and they're untrue! This sort of advertising just reinforces the images we get fed up about – having to look good, be thin and have good skin – and it's not fair!

I think it's essential to dispel the myths about the condition and educate people so they don't treat skin diseases as unimportant, let alone disgusting – or humorous – but with understanding and sympathy.

In terms of advice to other partners of people with acne, the key areas are to offer help and to be aware of what your partner wants. Talk if he or she wants to. Listen as long as it takes. And then don't dwell on the subject.

Don't focus on the spot, or the mark left by the spot – but focus on other things about them, to try to help them feel good, or better.

And it's important not to say they look good when they don't!

Don't say, 'it's not too bad' or 'it's not very noticeable.' This doesn't help at all – and is only annoying. The person with acne knows it doesn't look good and they want honesty.

If the acne looks bad, it's better to say so but with sympathy, 'Are you OK? – it looks bad, or painful.'

Sometimes it's better to say, 'I can see you're in pain, is there anything we can do about it? Get it out of the way between you so you can move on and get on with what you were doing.

Also, never say, 'I've had spots too, I know what it's like' – unless you also suffer from acne and really know what it's like.

There have been very low times for us both, but at the end of the day we're still together. We're both very aware of her acne – it's still a problem – it's not going to go away and you can't turn your back on it. But if you want to be together you just have to go on and work it through together.

The support an acne sufferer gets from a partner is important. Jill doesn't rely on me, but she knows we can talk about it together and it won't be dismissed.

12

The Outlook

Given that 80 per cent of all adolescents suffer from acne and that acne still affects 1 to 5 per cent of adults at the age of 40, we are dealing with a massive problem. If you audit doctor practice, however, you find that doctors see only very few patients with acne – so what happens to all those that do not seek medical advice?

It is obvious from the very inaccurate figures that are available, that fewer than 25 per cent of patients with acne seek medical advice. Many patients come for specialist treatment too late, with significant scarring of the skin already present. We know that anti-acne products which you can buy at the pharmacist can work in mild acne, but even taking this into account there are still thousands of sufferers who need proper medical treatment who do not ask for it.

Much of this is due to lack of information – many patients do not realize that effective treatment is available. Because of the force of advertising for anti-acne treatments, many people feel that if their acne fails to respond to these treatments – which they've been told will work – they are in some way abnormal and that their problem will not respond to *any* treatment.

The myth that you will always grow out of acne also makes patients complacent – 'I won't bother the doctor, as it's going to get better by itself anyway.' That may be true for some, but may not be true for you!

What we need is a change in society's view on acne, so that the problem is taken seriously and support and effective treatment are offered. We need to educate the public of all ages about the cause of acne and the treatments that are available, to empower people to get the best that modern medicine can offer. These are some of the goals of the Acne Support Group, and hopefully this book will go some way towards helping to achieve them.

Lack of information or poor and confusing information is an important factor in the low uptake of medical treatment of acne. However, lack of knowledge by doctors must significantly contribute to this. Most doctors have only three to four weeks of training in skin medicine during their medical education. This does not provide sufficient expertise to manage all the skin problems that a normal doctor has to deal with. Up to 10 per cent of visits to a doctor are about a skin problem. Postgraduate training in skin diseases for doctors is becoming more common, but many doctors are still poorly prepared to deal with patients with difficult acne.

What about the dermatologist? There are only about 300 dermatologists in the UK, serving a population of over 55 million. At present numbers, dermatologists can only provide a service for the most difficult skin problems.

The answer is to provide better training for doctors in skin diseases, provide further education for doctors once they have qualified, and increase the number of skin specialists available in the UK. Daunting tasks, to be sure, but ones that will never be achieved unless they are tackled. Pressure from patients is probably the most effective way of bringing about these changes.

From the medical standpoint, the future of acne looks good. Research has started to dissect the mechanisms underlying the development of acne, and this should lead to a more effective approach to management of this disease. We now know that the immune system is involved in the generation of the inflammatory response in acne, and this should lead to a new generation of anti-acne treatments.

There are a number of problems with existing anti-acne treatments which makes many of them less than optimal. What we need for the ideal treatment of acne is a drug that can be taken in tablet form and that reduces oil production in the skin, clears the partial blockage in the follicle and prevents it from recurring and stops the inflammatory response to *Propionibacterium acnes*, but has no side-effects and produces a cure with the first course of treatment. This is something to aim at, but something that we will not easily achieve. The closest we have come to this ideal is Roaccutane®, but this drug does have significant side-effects and is associated with significant relapse rates (*see Chapter 5*).

Antibiotics will reduce the inflammatory response, partly by their action on the immune response and partly by killing *Propionibacterium acnes*. Antibiotics can cause problems with side-effects, most of which are minor. Apart from minocycline, antibiotics used in acne are now associated with increasing resistance in the bacterial populations in the skin. Newer antibiotics are being evaluated which will hopefully give a broader range of drugs that we can use in acne.

Topical vitamin A derivatives will clear the partial blockage of the follicles and prevent their reformation, which will ultimately prevent new spots from developing. These agents are slow in their action and are often very irritating to the skin, which limits their use. Newer topical vitamin A derivatives such as Differin® are less irritating and better tolerated, and more are now being evaluated which may cause fewer side-effects and will be more acceptable to patients.

Although we still do not have the perfect treatment for acne, the range of treatments we do have available will provide effective control of acne in the vast majority of patients.

The treatments are there. If you do not ask for them, you will not get them. If doctors are not aware of them, they will not prescribe them.

It's Up to You!

You must take responsibility for your acne, seek advice and never be complacent – if things are not getting better, demand better treatment!

Useful Addresses

Acne Support Group
(for acne and rosacea sufferers)
PO Box 230
Hayes
Middlesex UB4 9HW
Tel/Fax: 0181 561 6868
Advice, support and information, relaxation tapes, etc.

Changing Faces
1 & 2 Junction Mews
London W2 1PN
Tel: 0171 706 4232
Fax: 0171 706 4234
For children and adults suffering facial disfigurement

Samaritans
National number: 0345 909090

Relate
Local branches listed in local telephone directories
National Office:
Herbert Gray College
Little Church Street
Rugby CV21 3AP
Tel: 01788 563816
Fax: 01788 552210
Relate-line Counselling 0870 601 2121 (Weekdays 9.30 a.m. –
1 p.m.)

Depression Alliance
PO Box 1022
London SE1 7QB
Tel: 0171 633 9929

Complementary Medicine

British Acupuncture Council
Park House
206–208 Latimer Road
London W10 6RE
Tel: 0181 964 0222

The Chi Centre
10 Greycoat Place
London SW1P 1SB
(affiliated to the Institute of Complementary Medicine)
Chi Helpline: 0171 222 1888

The Faculty of Homoeopathy
Hahnemann House
2 Powis Place
Great Ormond Street
London WC1N 3HT
Tel: 0171 837 9469

Further Reading

Leon Chaitow, *Candida Albicans* (Thorsons)

Dr Stephen T Chang, *The Complete System of Chinese Self-healing* (Thorsons)

Angela Hicks, *Principles of Acupuncture* (Thorsons)

Robert Holden, *Stress Busters* (Thorsons)

Tony Lake, *Defeating Depression* (Penguin)

Spike Milligan and Anthony Clare, *Depression and How to Survive It* (Arrow)

Dr Melvyn R Werbach, *Healing Through Nutrition* (Thorsons)

Other related titles are available by post from:

Relate Books With Care

Herbert Gray College

Little Church Street

Rugby CV21 3AP
Tel: 01788 563816
Fax: 01788 552210

Also books from the 'Self-esteem' booklist, such as:
Dr Paul Hauck, *Hold Your Head Up High* (Sheldon Press)
Fred Orr, *Conquering Shyness*

Glossary

Alpha hydroxyacids   These are acids derived from fruit and have been shown to be helpful in the treatment of acne.

Anaerobic   This means that the bacterium can only grow when there is no oxygen available. Such conditions are found within the hair follicle.

Azelaic acid   This is a drug that has an antibacterial effect but also has an effect on a microcomedone formation and will help to unblock hair follicles.

Benzoyl peroxide   This is the constituent of most of the anti-acne creams that you can buy at the pharmacist. It is an oxidizer and kills the bacteria by introducing oxygen into the follicle.

Blackheads   These are open comedones where blockage within the hair canal leads to the build-up of solidified oil within the canal. As the blockage is close to the surface, a mixture of pigment and oxidized oil forms a black colour which is the black of the blackhead.

Candida albicans   This is a yeast that is the cause of thrush.

Collagen   Collagen is a fibrous protein that is one of the building blocks of the body. There are several different types of collagen which are found in different organs of the body. In the skin the collagen forms the foundation of the skin within the dermis upon which the top layer of skin, or epidermis, rests. Collagen is produced in the skin by specialized cells called fibroblasts.

Cyproterone acetate   This is a progesterone hormone which reduces the effect of testosterone on the body.

Cyst   An acne cyst is composed of part of the hair follicle which has become detached and has rounded up, rather like a flattened balloon, within the deeper layers of the skin. This will accumulate cell debris and oil and will act as a focus for infection. When these cysts become infected they can become very large and extremely painful.

Dapsone   This is an anti-inflammatory drug which is used worldwide in the treatment of leprosy. It has an effect on inflammation and is used extensively in dermatology in a variety of diseases.

Dermis   This is the second and deeper part of the skin which is composed of collagen that supports the skin and contains blood vessels, nerves and other skin structures.

Dianette®   This is a treatment for acne that contains two hormones: one, the female hormone oestrogen, and the second, a drug called cyproterone acetate which counteracts testosterone.

Differin® gel   This contains a chemical that has a vitamin A like activity. (Not available in the US.)

Drug resistance   This is where bacteria are able to change their genetic make-up so that antibiotics can no longer harm them.

Epidermis   This is the topmost layer of the skin, composed of cells that continually grow. As the cells grow they mature and are eventually shed as dead skin scales.

Fibroblasts   This is the cell within the dermis which produces collagen.

Glucose-6-phosphate dehydrogenase   This is an enzyme present in red blood cells. Absence of this enzyme makes the blood cells more susceptible to the damaging effects of Dapsone.

Hepatitis   This is inflammation in the liver. It can be caused by infections, but a number of drugs can also cause hepatitis.

Isolutrol   This is a chemical that was originally extracted from Shark's bile but is now chemically synthesized. It is present in preparations that are reported to reduce oil production in the skin.

Isotretinoin   This is the chemical name for Roaccutane®.

Isotrex® gel   This is a vitamin A preparation. (Not available in the US.)

Keloid   This is a scar that has become thickened as the scar-producing cells have overgrown. Keloids are often itchy or painful.

Keratolytic   This effectively means dissolving dead skin. The top layer of the skin and the partial blockage that develops in the follicle in the development of acne are composed of dead skin cells. A keratolytic agent will dissolve these.

Microcomedone   This is the partial blockage that develops in the hair canal and is the pre-cursor of all acne lesions.

Oestrogen   This is the female hormone produced by the ovaries which counteracts testosterone.

Papule   This is the first inflamed spot of acne and presents as a slightly raised red bump on the skin. If the inflammation is deep, these can be painful or throb.

Pilosebaceous follicle   This is the unit composed of the hair follicle with its attached sebaceous gland. This is the site at which acne occurs.

Pitted scarring   Pitted scarring is caused by loss of part of the dermis such that a dimple occurs in the skin or the epidermis is pulled down into the dermis causing an ice pick-like scar.

Porphyrins   These are chemicals that are excited by certain wavelengths of light. Porphyrins are present in the bacterium, *Propionibacterium acnes*, known to be the cause of the inflammatory lesions of acne.

Progesterone   This is a female hormone produced by the ovaries. Some progesterones can be metabolized in the liver to produce male hormone-like hormones.

Propionibacterium acnes   This is a bacterium found within the hair follicle that is thought to be the major cause of the inflammatory lesions of acne.

Pustule   This is a spot filled with pus and is one of the late-stage acne spots.

Retin A®   This is a vitamin A derivative which is made up in either a gel, cream or lotion formulation.

Retinoid   This is a drug with a vitamin A-like activity.

Roaccutane®   This is an orally active form of vitamin A that is used in the treatment of severe acne.

Salicylic acid   This is the main constituent of aspirin. Salicylic acid when used on the skin will dissolve dead skin cells and is therefore keratolytic.

Sebaceous gland   This is the gland which is attached to the hair follicle and produces oil in response to the male

hormone testosterone, and also in response to ambient
temperature.

Sebum   This is the mixture of oil produced by the sebaceous
gland that is pumped by the hair follicle and by the skin
pore onto the surface of the skin.

Spironolactone   This drug is a diuretic – that is, a drug
that makes you pass more urine – which has the effect of
blocking the male hormone.

Testosterone   This is the male hormone which is produced in
men in the testes and in women by the adrenal glands and
ovaries.

Tetracyclines   This is a class of antibiotic drug that includes
tetracycline, oxytetracycline, Minocin®, minocycline,
doxycycline, Vibramycin®, and lymecycline.

Ultraviolet light   This is low wavelength sunlight which
causes tanning of the skin and sunburn.

Venous thrombosis   This is the development of clots within
the veins, usually in the legs.

Whitehead   This is a deep comedone in which the blockage
is deep within the epidermis and therefore is not visible
from the surface. The build-up of solidified oil within the
follicle pushes the skin up as a small raised bump.

Index